Echo
Made Easy

SECOND EDITION

Sam Kaddoura

BSc(Hons), BM BCh(Oxon), PhD, DIC, FRCP, FESC, FACC

Consultant Cardiologist,
Chelsea and Westminster Hospital and Royal Brompton Hospital,
London
Honorary Consultant Cardiologist,
Royal Hospital Chelsea, London
Honorary Senior Lecturer,
Imperial College School of Medicine, London, UK

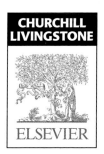

Edinburgh   London   New York   Oxford   Philadelphia   St Louis   Sydney   Toronto   2009

CHURCHILL LIVINGSTONE
ELSEVIER

© 2002, Elsevier Limited.
© 2009, Sam Kaddoura. All rights reserved.

The right of Sam Kaddoura to be identified as author of this work has been asserted by him in accordance with the Copyright, Design and Patents Act 1988.

First published 2002
Second edition 2009

Main edition ISBN: 978-0-443-10363-6
International Edition ISBN: 978-0-443-10364-3

British Library Cataloguing in Publication Data
A catalogue record for this book is available from the British Library

Library of Congress Cataloging in Publication Data
A catalog record for this book is available from the Library of Congress

Notice
Knowledge and best practice in this field are constantly changing. As new research and experience broaden our knowledge, changes in practice, treatment and drug therapy may become necessary or appropriate. Readers are advised to check the most current information provided (i) on procedures featured or (ii) by the manufacturer of each product to be administered, to verify the recommended dose or formula, the method and duration of administration, and contraindications. It is the responsibility of the practitioner, relying on their own experience and knowledge of the patient, to make diagnoses, to determine dosages and the best treatment for each individual patient, and to take all appropriate safety precautions. To the fullest extent of the law, neither the Publisher nor the Author assumes any liability for any injury and/or damage to persons or property arising out or related to any use of the material contained in this book.

The Publisher

ELSEVIER your source for books, journals and multimedia in the health sciences

www.elsevierhealth.com

Working together to grow
libraries in developing countries

www.elsevier.com | www.bookaid.org | www.sabre.org

ELSEVIER   BOOK AID International   Sabre Foundation

The publisher's policy is to use **paper manufactured from sustainable forests**

Printed in China

Preface

Echocardiography (echo) is the use of ultrasound to examine the heart. It is a powerful and safe technique which has become widely available for cardiovascular investigation. The training of medical students and newly qualified doctors often includes an introduction to echo. Undergraduate and postgraduate examinations such as MRCP (UK) sometimes set questions on the subject.

While there are many detailed texts of echo available, aimed primarily at cardiologists and those performing echo examinations, such as cardiac technicians, there are few simply introductory texts.

This book aims to provide a practical and clinically useful introduction to echo – much of which *is* easy – for those who will be using, requesting and possibly interpreting it in the future. The book is aimed particularly at doctors in training and medical students. It is also hoped that it may be of interest to other groups – established physicians, surgeons and general practitioners, cardiac technicians, nurses and paramedics.

It aims to explain the echo techniques available, what an echo can and can't give, and – importantly – puts echo into a clinical perspective. It is by no means intended as a complete textbook of echo and some aspects are far beyond its scope (e.g. complex congenital heart disease and paediatric echo).

This new edition has become necessary because of advances in echocardiography over the past six years. New sections have been added on device therapy for heart failure (cardiac resynchronization therapy, CRT) and the use of echo and transoesophageal echo (TOE or TEE) in special situations such as intraoperatively and in critically ill patients. The section on diastolic function has been expanded with the addition of tissue Doppler imaging, and the section on pericardial disease has been made more detailed. There are expanded sections on newer echo techniques such as 3-D echo, stress echo and contrast echo and a new section on pulmonary embolism. Special clinical situations now include echo changes with advanced age, the athletic heart, obesity and diet drugs.

The aim has been to keep the book around the same length as the previous edition, but inevitably there has been some increase due to new figures and text. Full colour illustrations are used throughout for this new edition.

Sam Kaddoura
London
2008

Acknowledgements

I am grateful to Professor A. R. Kaddoura and Dr N. Shamaa for their enormous help in the preparation of the book. I also should like to thank Dr Phil Carrillo, Dr Gerry Carr-White, Dr Michael Henein, Dr Rohan Jagathesan, Mrs Johan Carberry, Mrs Myrtle Crathern, Mrs Renomee Porten, Mrs Sonia Williams, Dr Sanjay Prasad, Mrs Denise Udo and Dr Ihab Ramzy. I am also very grateful to Miss Natalie McDonnell, Dr Jamil Mayet, Dr Rakesh Sharma, Dr Wei Li, Miss Beth Unsworth and Mr Graham Clark. Last but not least, many thanks to Mrs Janice Urquhart, Ms Christine Johnston and Mr Laurence Hunter of Elsevier for their support and patience!

Contents

Abbreviations

A_2	Aortic second heart sound	3-D	Three-dimensional echocardiography
ACE	Angiotensin-converting enzyme		
AF	Atrial fibrillation	E-wave	Early wave of mitral flow
A_m	Atrial myocardial velocity	ECG	Electrocardiograph
AMVL	Anterior mitral valve leaflet	Echo	Echocardiography/echocardiogram
Ao	Aorta		
AR	Aortic regurgitation	EF	Ejection fraction
AS	Aortic stenosis	E_m	Early myocardial velocity
ASD	Atrial septal defect	EMD	Electro-mechanical delay
ASH	Asymmetrical septal hypertrophy	EPS	Electrophysiological study
		ESR	Erythrocyte sedimentation rate
AT	Acceleration time		
AV	Aortic valve	FS	Fractional shortening
A-wave	Atrial wave of mitral flow	FVI	Flow velocity integral
BART	Blue away, red towards	HCM	Hypertrophic cardiomyopathy
BP	Blood pressure	HF	Heart failure
BSA	Body surface area	HOCM	Hypertrophic obstructive cardiomyopathy
CABG	Coronary artery bypass grafting	5-HT	5-Hydroxytryptamine
CF	Colour flow	IAS	Interatrial septum
CRT	Cardiac resynchronization therapy	IE	Infective endocarditis
		ITU	Intensive therapy unit
CRT-D	Cardiac resynchronization therapy – defibrillator	i.v.	Intravenous
		IVC	Inferior vena cava
CRT-P	Cardiac resynchronization therapy – pacemaker	IVRT	Isovolumic relaxation time
CSA	Cross-sectional area	IVS	Interventricular septum
CT	Computed tomography	JVP	Jugular venous pressure
CVA	Cerebrovascular accident		
CW	Continuous wave	LA	Left atrium
		LBBB	Left bundle branch block
DT	Deceleration time	LV	Left ventricle
2-D	Two-dimensional echocardiography	LVEDD	Left ventricular end-diastolic diameter

LVEF	Left ventricular ejection fraction	PV	Pulmonary valve
LVESD	Left ventricular end-systolic diameter	PW	Pulsed wave
LVH	Left ventricular hypertrophy	RA	Right atrium
LVOT	Left ventricular outflow tract	RAP	Right atrial pressure
LVOTO	Left ventricular outflow tract obstruction	RBBB	Right bundle branch block
		RV	Right ventricle
LVPW	Left ventricular posterior wall	RVSP	Right ventricular systolic pressure
MI	Myocardial infarction	RVOT	Right ventricular outflow tract
MR	Mitral regurgitation	RVOTO	Right ventricular outflow tract obstruction
MRI	Magnetic resonance imaging		
MS	Mitral stenosis	S_1, S_2, etc.	First, second heart sounds, etc.
M-mode	Motion-mode	SAM	Systolic anterior motion
MV	Mitral valve	SBE	Subacute bacterial endocarditis
		SLE	Systemic lupus erythematosus
NYHA	New York Heart Association	SVt	Supraventricular tachycardia
P_2	Pulmonary second sound	TDI	Tissue Doppler imaging
ΔP	Pressure gradient	TIA	Transient ischaemic attack
PA	Pulmonary artery	TOE/TEE	Transoesophageal echocardiography
PASP	Pulmonary artery systolic pressure	TR	Tricuspid regurgitation
PCI	Percutaneous coronary intervention	TS	Tricuspid stenosis
PDA	Patent ductus arteriosus	TTE	Transthoracic echocardiography
PE	Pulmonary embolism	TV	Tricuspid valve
PFO	Patent foramen ovale		
PHT	Pulmonary hypertension	V	Velocity
PMVL	Posterior mitral valve leaflet	VF	Ventricular fibrillation
PR	Pulmonary regurgitation	VSD	Ventricular septal defect
PS	Pulmonary stenosis	VT	Ventricular tachycardia

CHAPTER 1

What is echo?

1.1 BASIC NOTIONS

Echocardiography (echo) – the use of ultrasound to examine the heart – is a safe, powerful, non-invasive and painless technique.

Echo is easy to understand as many features are based upon simple physical and physiological facts. It is a practical procedure requiring skill and is very operator dependent – the quality of the echo study and the information derived from it are influenced by who carries out the examination!

This chapter deals with:

- Ultrasound production and detection
- The echo techniques in common clinical use
- The normal echo
- Who should have an echo.

Ultrasound production and detection

Sound is a disturbance propagating in a material – air, water, body tissue or a solid substance. Each sound is characterized by its frequency and its intensity. Frequency is measured in hertz (Hz), i.e. in oscillations per second, and its multiples (kilohertz, kHz, 10^3 Hz and megahertz, MHz, 10^6 Hz). Sound of frequency higher than 20 kHz cannot be perceived by the human ear and is called ultrasound. Echo uses ultrasound of frequencies ranging from about 1.5 MHz to about 7.5 MHz. The nature of the material in which the sound propagates determines its velocity. In the heart, the velocity is 1540 m/s. The speed of sound in air is 330 m/s.

The wavelength of sound equals the ratio of velocity to frequency. In heart tissue, ultrasound with a frequency of 5 MHz has a wavelength of about 0.3 mm. The shorter the wavelength, the higher the resolution. As a rough estimate, the smallest size that can be resolved by a sound is equal to its wavelength. On the other hand, the smaller the wavelength of the sound, the less its penetration power. So a compromise has to be struck between resolution and penetration. A higher frequency of ultrasound can be used in children since less depth of penetration is needed.

Ultrasound results from the property of certain crystals to transform electrical oscillations (varying voltages) into mechanical oscillations (sound). This is called the piezoelectric effect (Fig. 1.1). The same crystals can also act as ultrasound receivers since they can effect the transformation in the opposite direction (mechanical to electrical).

The repetition rate is 1000/second. Each transmitting and receiving period lasts for 1 ms. Transmission accounts for 1 µs of this time. The remaining time is spent in 'receiving' mode.

At the core of any echo machine is this piezoelectric crystal transducer. When varying voltages are applied to the crystal, it vibrates and transmits ultrasound. When the crystal is in receiving mode, if it is struck by ultrasound waves, it is distorted. This generates an electrical signal which is analysed by the echo machine. The crystal can receive as long as it is not transmitting at that time. This fixes the function of the crystal – it emits a pulse and then listens for a reflection.

When ultrasound propagates in a uniform medium, it maintains its initial direction and is progressively absorbed or scattered. If it meets a discontinuity such as the interface of 2 parts of the medium having different densities, some of the ultrasound is reflected back. Ultrasound meets many tissue interfaces and echo reflections occur from different depths. Some interfaces or tissues are more echo-reflective than others (e.g. bone or calcium are more reflective than blood) and these appear as echo-bright reflections.

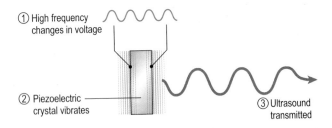

Fig. 1.1 *Piezoelectric effect.*

Two quantities are measured in an echo:

1. The time delay between transmission of the pulse and reception of the reflected echo
2. The intensity of the reflected signal, indicating the echo-reflectivity of that tissue or tissue–tissue interface.

The signals that return to the transducer therefore give evidence of depth and intensity of reflection. These are transformed electronically into greyscale images on a TV screen or printed on paper – high echo reflection is white, less reflection is grey and no reflection is black.

1.2 VIEWING THE HEART

Echo studies are carried out using specialized ultrasound machines. Ultrasound of different frequencies (in adults usually 2–4 MHz) is transmitted from a transducer (probe) which is placed on the subject's anterior chest wall. This is transthoracic echo (TTE). The transducer usually has a line or dot to help rotate it into the correct position to give different echo views. The subject usually lies in the left lateral position and ultrasound jelly is placed on the transducer to ensure good images. Continuous electrocardiograph (ECG) recording is performed and phonocardiography may be used to time cardiac events. An echo examination usually takes 15–20 min.

Echo 'windows' and views (Fig. 1.2)

There are a number of standard positions on the chest wall for the transducer where there are 'echo windows' that allow good penetration by ultrasound without too much masking and absorption by lung or ribs.

A number of sections of the heart are examined by echo from these transducer positions, which are used for 2 main reasons:

1. There is a limitation determined by the anatomy of the heart and its surrounding structures
2. To produce standardized images that can be compared between different studies.

Useful echo information can be obtained in most subjects, but the study can be technically difficult in:

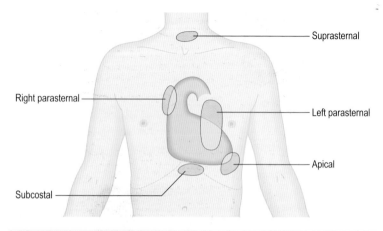

Fig. 1.2 *The main echo 'windows'.*

- Very obese subjects
- Those with chest wall deformities
- Those with chronic lung disease (e.g. chronic airflow limitation with hyperinflated lungs or pulmonary fibrosis).

Rarely, an echo study is impossible.

A number of 'echo views' are obtained in most studies. 'Axis' refers to the plane in which the ultrasound beam travels through the heart.

Left parasternal window. (2nd–4th intercostal space, left sternal edge):

1. **Long-axis view** (Figs 1.3, 1.4). Most examinations begin with this view. The transducer is used to obtain images of the heart in long axis, with slices from the base of the heart to the apex. The marker dot on the transducer points to the right shoulder.

2. **Short-axis views** (Figs 1.5, 1.6). Without moving the transducer from its location on the chest wall and by rotating the transducer through 90° so the marker dot is pointing towards the left shoulder, the heart is cut in transverse (short-axis) sections. By changing the angulation on the chest wall, it is possible to obtain any number of short-axis views, but the standard 4 are at the level of the aortic valve (AV), mitral valve (MV), left ventricular papillary muscles and left ventricular apex (Figs 1.5, 1.6).

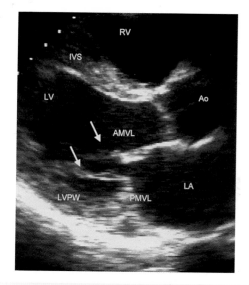

Fig. 1.3 *Parasternal long-axis view. Arrows show chordae.*

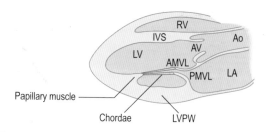

Fig. 1.4 *Parasternal long-axis view.*

Apical window. (Cardiac apex):

1. **4-chamber view** (Figs 1.7a, 1.8a). The transducer is placed at the cardiac apex with the marker dot pointing down towards the left shoulder. This gives the typical 'heart-shaped' 4-chamber view (Fig. 1.7a).

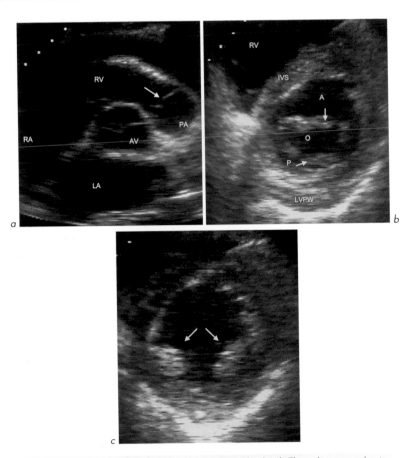

Fig. 1.5 *Parasternal short-axis views:* **(a)** *Aortic valve level. The pulmonary valve is shown (arrow).* **(b)** *Mitral valve level. The anterior (A) and posterior (P) leaflets are shown. Mitral orifice (O).* **(c)** *Papillary muscles (arrows) level.*

2. **5-chamber (including aortic outflow)** (Figs 1.7b, 1.8b). By altering the angulation of the transducer so the ultrasound beam is angled more anteriorly towards the chest wall, a '5-chamber' view is obtained. The 5th 'chamber' is not a chamber at all but is the AV and ascending aorta. This is useful in assessing aortic stenosis (AS) and aortic regurgitation (AR).

Parasternal short-axis views

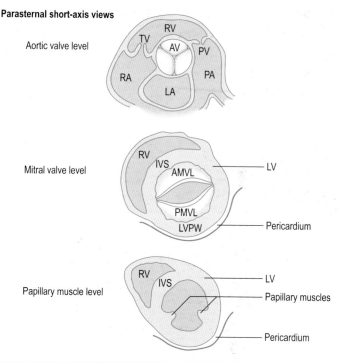

Fig. 1.6 *Parasternal short-axis views.*

3. **Long-axis and 2-chamber views** (Figs 1.7c, 1.8c). By rotating the transducer on the cardiac apex it is possible to obtain apical long-axis and 2-chamber views which show different segments of the left ventricle (LV).

Subcostal window. (Under the xiphisternum) (Fig. 1.9):
Similar views to apical views, but rotated by 90°. Useful in lung disease, for imaging the interatrial septum, inferior vena cava (IVC) and abdominal aorta.

Further windows may be used:

Suprasternal window. (For imaging the aorta in coarctation).

Right parasternal window. (In AS and to examine the ascending aorta).

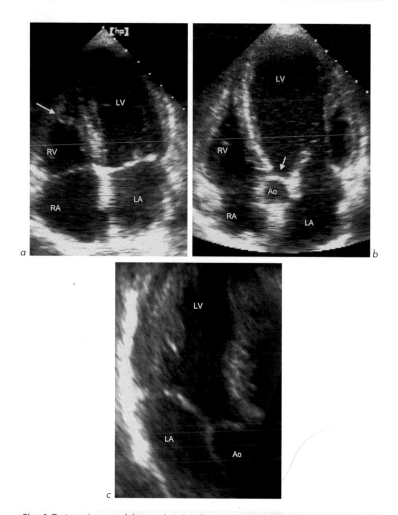

Fig. 1.7 Apical views: **(a)** Apical 4-chamber view. A moderator band is shown (arrow). This is a normal neuromuscular bundle carrying right bundle branch fibres. **(b)** Apical 5-chamber view. The aortic valve is shown (arrow). **(c)** Apical long-axis view.

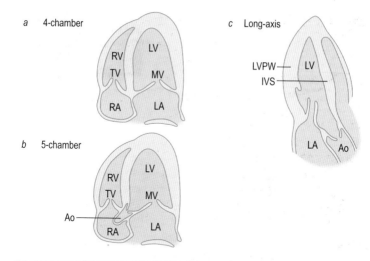

a 4-chamber

b 5-chamber

c Long-axis

Fig. 1.8 Apical views.

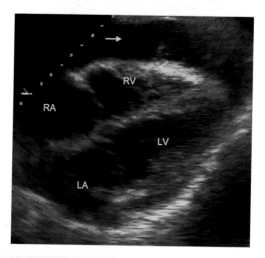

Fig. 1.9 Subcostal 4-chamber view. A pericardial effusion is seen (arrow).

1.3 ECHO TECHNIQUES

Three echo methods are in common clinical usage:

- Two-dimensional (2-D) or 'cross-sectional'
- Motion or M-mode
- Doppler – continuous wave, pulsed wave and colour flow.

2-D echo gives a snapshot in time of a cross-section of tissue. If these sections are produced in quick succession and displayed on a TV screen, they can show 'real-time imaging' of the heart chambers, valves and blood vessels.

To create a 2-D image, the ultrasound beam must be swept across the area of interest. The transducer rotates the beam it produces through a certain angle, either mechanically or electronically (Fig. 1.10). In the first case, the transducer is rotated so that its beam scans the target. In the second case, several crystals are mounted together and are excited by voltages in sequence. Each crystal emits waves. The result is a summation wave which moves in a direction determined

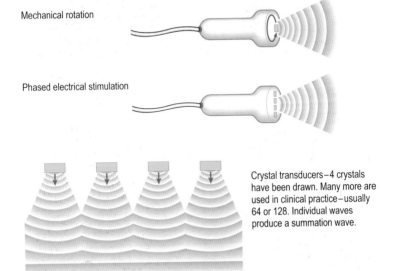

Mechanical rotation

Phased electrical stimulation

Crystal transducers – 4 crystals have been drawn. Many more are used in clinical practice – usually 64 or 128. Individual waves produce a summation wave.

Fig. 1.10 *Mechanical and electronic transducers.*

by the 'phased stimulation' of the crystals. The reflected ultrasound generates an electrical signal in the crystal, which is used to produce a dot on the TV screen. Ultrasound is transmitted along scan lines (usually about 120 lines) over an arc of approximately 90° at least 20–30 times per second and in some newer systems up to 120 times per second. Reflected ultrasound signals are combined on the TV screen to build up a moving image. Frozen images can be printed out on paper or photographic film.

Motion or M-mode echo (Fig. 1.11) is produced by the transmission and reception of an ultrasound signal along only one line, giving high sensitivity

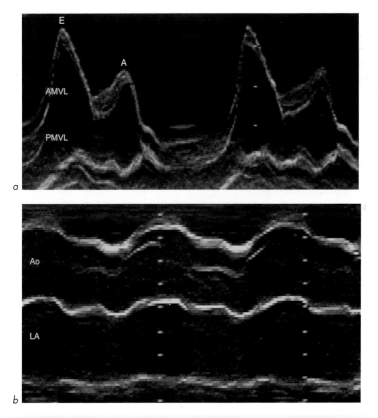

Fig. 1.11 *M-mode patterns. (a) Mitral valve and (b) aortic root and left atrium.*

(greater than 2-D echo) for recording moving structures. It produces a graph of depth and strength of reflection with time. Changes in movement (e.g. valve opening and closing or ventricular wall movement) can be displayed. The ultrasound signal should be aligned perpendicularly to the structure being examined. Measurement of the size and thickness of cardiac chambers can be made either manually on paper printouts or on the TV screen using computer software.

Doppler echo uses the reflection of ultrasound by moving red blood cells. The Doppler principle is used to derive velocity information (Ch. 3). The reflected ultrasound has a frequency shift relative to the transmitted ultrasound, determined by the velocity and direction of blood flow. This gives haemodynamic information regarding the heart and blood vessels. It can be used to measure the severity of valvular narrowing (stenosis), to detect valvular leakage (regurgitation) and can show intracardiac shunts such as ventricular septal defects (VSDs) and atrial septal defects (ASDs) (Ch. 6). The 3 commonly used Doppler echo techniques are:

1. **Continuous wave Doppler.** Two crystals are used – one transmitting continuously and one receiving continuously. This technique is useful for measuring high velocities but its ability to localize a flow signal precisely is limited since the signal can originate at any point along the length or width of the ultrasound beam (Fig. 1.12).

2. **Pulsed wave Doppler** (Fig. 1.13). This allows a flow disturbance to be localized or blood velocity from a small region to be measured. A single crystal is used to transmit an ultrasound signal and then to receive after a pre-set time delay. Reflected signals are only recorded from a depth corresponding to half the product of the time delay and the speed of sound in tissues (1540 m/s). By combining this technique with 2-D imaging, a small 'sample volume' can be identified on the screen showing the region where velocities are being measured. The operator can move the sample volume. Because the time delay limits the rate at which sampling can occur, there is a limit to the maximum velocity that can be accurately detected, before a phenomenon known as 'aliasing' occurs, usually at velocities in excess of 2 m/s. The theoretical limit of the sampling rate is known as the Nyquist limit.

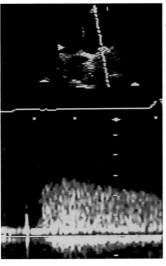

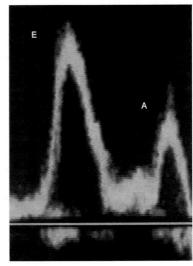

Fig. 1.12   Fig. 1.13

Fig. 1.12 *Continuous wave Doppler of severe mitral stenosis. Mean gradient 20 mmHg.*

Fig. 1.13 *Pulsed wave Doppler. Normal mitral flow pattern.*

Continuous wave and pulsed wave Doppler allow a graphical representation of velocity against time and are also referred to as 'spectral Doppler'.

3. **Colour flow mapping.** This is an automated 2-D version of pulsed wave Doppler. It calculates blood velocity and direction at multiple points along a number of scan lines superimposed on a 2-D echo image. The velocities and directions of blood flow are colour-encoded. Velocities away from the transducer are in blue, those towards it in red. This is known as the BART convention (Blue Away, Red Towards). Higher velocities are shown in progressively lighter shades of colour. Above a threshold velocity, 'colour reversal' occurs (explained again by the phenomenon of aliasing). Areas of high turbulence or regions of high flow acceleration are often indicated in green (Fig. 1.14).

13

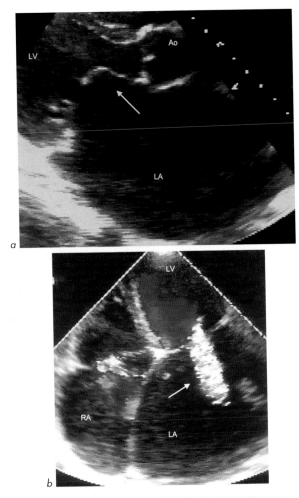

Fig. 1.14 *Rheumatic mitral regurgitation and stenosis. The left atrium is very enlarged. (a) The anterior leaflet shows 'elbowing' (arrow) on parasternal long-axis view. (b) A jet of mitral regurgitation is seen (arrow) on colour flow mapping in the apical 4-chamber view.*

Summary of echo modalities and their main uses

2-D echo
- anatomy
- ventricular and valvular movement
- positioning for M-mode and Doppler echo

M-mode echo
- measurement of dimensions
- timing cardiac events

Pulsed wave Doppler
- normal valve flow patterns
- LV diastolic function
- stroke volume and cardiac output

Continuous wave Doppler
- severity of valvular stenosis
- severity of valvular regurgitation
- velocity of flow in shunts

Colour flow mapping
- assessment of regurgitation and shunts.

1.4 THE NORMAL ECHO

Echo provides a great deal of anatomical and haemodynamic information:
- Heart chamber size
- Chamber function (systolic and diastolic)
- Valvular motion and function
- Intracardiac and extracardiac masses and fluid collections
- Direction of blood flow and haemodynamic information (e.g. valvular stenosis and pressure gradients) by Doppler echo.

'Normal echo ranges'

It is important to remember that these 'normal ranges' vary with a number of factors. The frequently quoted values of, e.g. left atrial diameter or left ventricular cavity internal dimensions do not take this into account. Important factors which influence cardiac dimensions measured by echo are:
- Height
- Sex
- Age
- Physical training (athletes).

In general, values are higher in taller individuals, males and athletes.

Some correction for these factors can be made, e.g. in very tall individuals, by indexing the measurement to body surface area (BSA):

$$BSA\,(m^2) = \sqrt{\frac{height\,(cm) \times weight\,(kg)}{3600}}$$

Bearing these points in mind, it is useful to have an indication of some *approximate* echo-derived 'Normal values' for an adult:

Left ventricle			
Internal diameter	end-systolic		2.0–4.0 cm
	end-diastolic		3.5–5.6 cm
Wall thickness	(diastolic)	septum	0.6–1.2 cm
		posterior wall	0.6–1.2 cm
	(systolic)	septum	0.9–1.8 cm
		posterior wall	0.9–1.8 cm
Fractional shortening			30–45%
Ejection fraction			50–85%
Left atrium (LA)			
Diameter			2.0–4.0 cm
Aortic root			
Diameter			2.0–4.0 cm
Right ventricle (RV)			
Diameter (systolic–diastolic)			0.7–2.3 cm

Some other findings on echo may be normal:

1. Mild tricuspid and mitral regurgitation (MR) are found in many normal hearts.
2. Some degree of thickening of AV leaflets with ageing is normal without significant aortic stenosis.
3. Mitral annulus (ring) calcification is sometimes seen in older subjects. It is often of no consequence but may be misdiagnosed as a stenosed valve, a vegetation (inflammatory mass), thrombus (clot) or myxoma (cardiac tumour). It is important to examine the leaflets carefully. It may be associated with MR (Fig. 1.15).

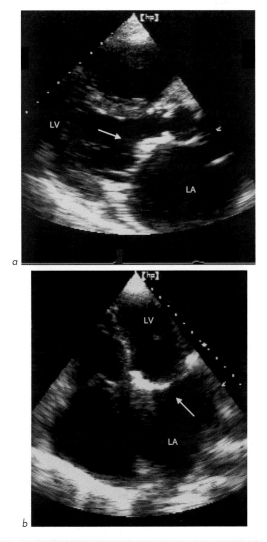

Fig. 1.15 Calcification of mitral annulus (arrow). This was asymptomatic, with no mitral stenosis or regurgitation. **(a)** Parasternal long-axis view. **(b)** Apical 4-chamber view.

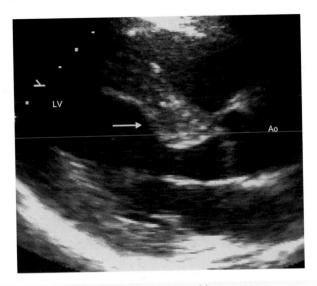

Fig. 1.16 *Upper septal bulge (arrow). Parasternal long-axis view.*

4. An 'upper septal bulge' (Fig. 1.16) is common, particularly in elderly women, and should not be misdiagnosed as hypertrophic cardiomyopathy (HCM). It is due to septal hypertrophy and fibrosis and only rarely causes significant LV outflow tract obstruction (LVOTO).

1.5 WHO SHOULD HAVE AN ECHO?

In order to obtain the most useful information, it is essential to provide:

- Adequate clinical information
- The reason an echo is being requested
- The specific question being asked.

Examples: '60-year-old man with breathlessness and previous anterior myocardial infarction, awaiting general anaesthesia for elective hip replacement surgery – please assess LV systolic function', or, '70-year-old woman with aortic ejection systolic murmur – please assess severity of aortic stenosis.'

The following list of indications is not exhaustive and others are found in the relevant sections of the book. The list gives situations in which an echo may influence the clinical management of a patient:

- Assessment of valve function, e.g. systolic or diastolic murmur
- Assessment of left ventricular function – systolic, diastolic and regional wall motion, e.g. suspected heart failure in a subject with breathlessness or oedema, or preoperative assessment
- Suspected endocarditis
- Suspected myocarditis
- Cardiac tamponade
- Pericardial disease (e.g. pericarditis) or pericardial effusion, especially if clinical evidence of tamponade
- Complications of myocardial infarction (MI), e.g. VSD, MR, effusion
- Suspicion of intracardiac masses – tumour, thrombus
- Cardiac chamber size, e.g. LA in atrial fibrillation (AF), cardiomegaly on chest X-ray
- Assessment of artificial (prosthetic) valve function
- Arrhythmias, e.g. AF, ventricular tachycardia (VT)
- Assessment of RV and right heart
- Estimation of intracardiac and vascular pressures, e.g. pulmonary artery systolic pressure (PASP) in lung disease and suspected pulmonary hypertension (PHT)
- Stroke and transient ischaemic attack (TIA) – 'cardiac source of embolism?'
- Exclusion of left ventricular hypertrophy (LVH) in hypertension
- Assessment of congenital heart disease.

1.6 MURMURS

A murmur is a sound caused by turbulent blood flow. It may be caused by:

- High velocity or volume across a normal valve
- Forward flow across a diseased valve
- Leakage across a valve
- Flow through a shunt (an abnormal communication between chambers or vessels)
- Flow across a narrowed blood vessel.

Echo helps to diagnose the underlying cause of a murmur and the severity of the haemodynamic effect, and to plan treatment.

1. Possible causes of a systolic murmur

- Benign flow murmur – features suggesting this are short, ejection, midsystolic, soft or moderate in loudness, normal second heart sound, may be louder on inspiration or on lying flat
- Aortic – 'sclerosis' or stenosis
- HCM
- Mitral – regurgitation, prolapse
- Pulmonary – stenosis
- Tricuspid – regurgitation (rarely heard – diagnosis made by seeing systolic waves in jugular venous pressure (JVP))
- Shunts – intracardiac or extracardiac – congenital, e.g. ASD (high flow across pulmonary valve (PV)), VSD, patent ductus arteriosus (PDA) or acquired (e.g. post-MI VSD)
- Coarctation of the aorta.

2. Conditions associated with a benign systolic murmur

(NO underlying cardiac disease) – common in childhood and pregnancy.

- Pulmonary flow – common, especially in young children (30%)
- Venous hum – continuous, reduced by neck vein compression, turning head laterally, bending elbows or lying down. Loudest in neck and around clavicles
- Mammary souffle – particularly in pregnancy
- High-flow states – pregnancy, anaemia, fever, anxiety, thyrotoxicosis (although in the case of thyrotoxicosis there may be associated cardiac disease).

3. Possible causes of a diastolic murmur

Abnormal – except venous hum or mammary souffle:
- Aortic – regurgitation
- Mitral – stenosis
- Pulmonary – regurgitation

- Tricuspid – stenosis (rare)
- Congenital shunts – e.g. PDA.

4. Who with a murmur should have an echo?

Features suggesting a murmur is pathological/organic

An echo should be requested for anyone whose murmur is not clearly clinically benign (e.g. pulmonary flow, venous hum, mammary souffle), especially if there are any features of a pathological murmur:

- Symptoms – chest pain, breathlessness, oedema, syncope, dizziness, palpitations
- Cyanosis
- Thrill (palpable murmur)
- Diastolic murmur*
- Pansystolic*
- Very loud murmur (but remember – the *loudness* of a murmur often bears no relation to the *severity* of the valve lesion)
- Added/abnormal heart sounds – abnormal S_2, ejection clicks, opening snaps, S_4 (not S_3 which can be normal, particularly if age <30 years)
- Physical signs of heart failure
- Wide pulse pressure and displaced apex
- Suspected endocarditis
- Suspected aortic dissection
- Cardiomegaly (e.g. on chest X-ray)
- Associated ECG abnormalities, e.g. LVH

(*exceptions are venous hum or mammary souffle as above)

CHAPTER 2

Valves

2.1 MITRAL VALVE (MV)

One of the earliest applications of echo was in the diagnosis of valvular heart disease, particularly mitral stenosis (MS). M-mode echo still provides very useful information, nowadays complemented by 2-D and Doppler techniques.

The MV is located between the LA and LV. The MV opens during ventricular diastole when blood flows from LA into LV. During ventricular systole, the MV closes as blood is ejected through the AV.

The MV has 3 main components:
- Leaflets (2) – anterior and posterior
- Chordae attached to papillary muscles ('subvalvular apparatus')
- Annulus (valve ring).

The 2 leaflets are attached at one end to the annulus and at the other (free) edge to the chordae which are fixed to the LV by the papillary muscles. The chordae hold each of the MV leaflets like cords hold a parachute canopy. The leaflets' free edges meet at 2 points called the commissures (Figs 2.1, 2.2).

Movement of the MV leaflets can be seen by M-mode and 2-D echo. The normal MV leaflets have a characteristic movement pattern on M-mode examination. The anterior MV leaflet (AMVL) sweeps an M-shape pattern, while the posterior leaflet (PMVL) sweeps a W-shaped pattern (Fig. 1.11a). Understanding the origin of the normal MV opening and closing pattern is easy and helps in understanding abnormal patterns in disease (Fig. 2.3).

The first peak of MV movement (early, E-wave) coincides with passive LA to LV flow. The second peak coincides with atrial contraction and active flow of blood into the LV (atrial, A-wave). This pattern of movement is brought about by the characteristics of blood flow into the LV. This second peak is lost in AF, where atrial mechanical activity is absent. On 2-D examination, the normal MV leaflets should be seen to be thin, mobile and separate and close well. Their motion should be of a double waveform as expected from the M-mode findings.

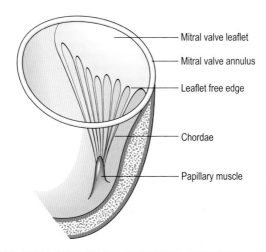

Fig. 2.1 *Attachment of one of the mitral valve leaflets.*

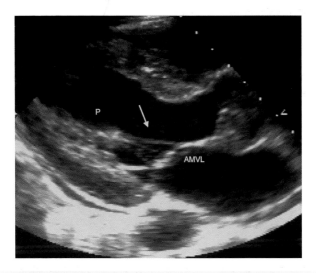

Fig. 2.2 *Part of the mitral valve apparatus. Anterior mitral valve leaflet, papillary muscle (P) and chordae tendineae (arrow).*

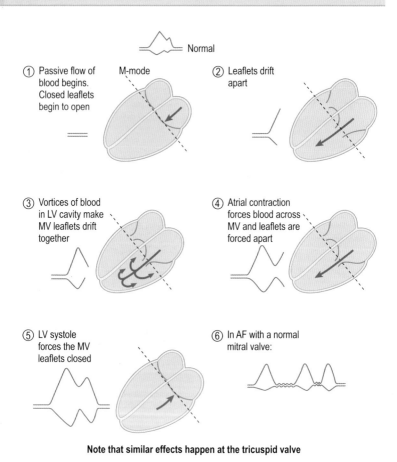

Note that similar effects happen at the tricuspid valve

Fig. 2.3 Origin of the M-mode pattern of normal mitral valve opening and closing.

The Doppler pattern of mitral flow shows a similar pattern to M-mode movement of the MV leaflets.

Mitral stenosis (MS)

In practical terms, the only common cause of MS is **rheumatic heart disease.**

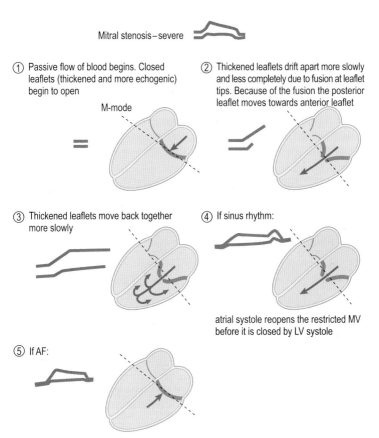

Mitral stenosis – severe

① Passive flow of blood begins. Closed leaflets (thickened and more echogenic) begin to open

② Thickened leaflets drift apart more slowly and less completely due to fusion at leaflet tips. Because of the fusion the posterior leaflet moves towards anterior leaflet

M-mode

③ Thickened leaflets move back together more slowly

④ If sinus rhythm:

atrial systole reopens the restricted MV before it is closed by LV systole

⑤ If AF:

Fig. 2.4 *Mitral stenosis – severe.*

Much rarer causes include mitral annulus calcification (usually asymptomatic and more likely to be associated with MR, rarely stenosis), congenital (may be associated with congenital aortic stenosis or aortic coarctation), connective tissue disorders and infiltrations, systemic lupus erythematosus (SLE), rheumatoid arthritis, mucopolysaccharidoses (Hurler's syndrome) and carcinoid.

Rheumatic fever is an autoimmune phenomenon caused by cross-reaction of antibodies to streptococcal bacterial antigens with antigens found on the heart.

In its acute stages, rheumatic fever is associated with inflammation of all layers of the heart – endocardium (including that of the valves), myocardium and pericardium. MS does not occur at this stage, but many years later as a consequence of this initial inflammatory process. The MV leaflets progressively fuse, initially at the commissures and free edges, which become thickened and later calcified. The inflamed valve becomes progressively thickened, fibrosed and calcified. This restricts the opening and closing of the valve. The chordae may also become thickened, shortened and calcified, further restricting normal valve function. The leaflets shrink and become rigid. The size of the MV orifice reduces leading to MS, which restricts blood flow from LA to LV.

Remember that many years elapse between rheumatic fever and the clinical manifestations of MS but there may not be a clear clinical history of rheumatic fever in childhood. Some individuals may remember being placed on bedrest for many weeks, which was the often-favoured treatment for rheumatic fever.

The **M-mode** pattern changes in a predictable way (Fig. 2.4). The movement of the leaflets is more restricted, and the leaflet tips are fused, so the posterior leaflet is pulled towards the anterior leaflet rather than drifting away from it. In severe MS, there is often AF rather than sinus rhythm, and the 2nd peak of MV movement is lost. The calcified leaflets reflect ultrasound in a different pattern from normal leaflets due to their increased thickness, fibrosis and often calcification. Instead of a single echo reflection giving a sharp image of the leaflets, there is a reverberation with several echo reflections giving a fuzzy image. Calcified leaflets produce a stronger echo reflection.

On **2-D echo**, the MV leaflets can be seen to be thickened and their movement restricted. Because of the fusion of the anterior and posterior leaflet tips, while the leaflet cusps may remain relatively mobile, there may be a characteristic 'elbowing' or 'bent-knee' appearance, particularly of the anterior MV leaflet (Figs 2.5, 2.6). This has also been likened to the bulging of a boat's sail as it fills with wind. The LA also enlarges.

The computer of the echo machine can calculate the area of the MV orifice after tracing around a frozen image on a parasternal short-axis view taken at the level of the MV leaflets in end-diastole. The normal leaflets in this view can be seen to open and close in a 'fish-mouth' pattern. In MS, the leaflet tips are calcified and opening is restricted with a reduced orifice size.

MV orifice area (Fig. 2.7) can also be measured using Doppler (Ch. 3).

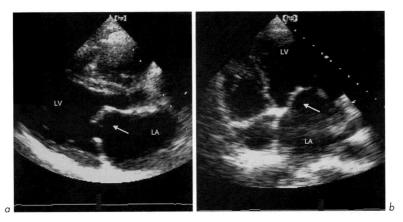

Fig. 2.5 *Rheumatic mitral stenosis. (a) Parasternal long-axis view and (b) apical 4-chamber view. 'Elbowing' of the anterior mitral valve leaflet is shown (arrow).*

Changes in MV area with severity of MS

- Normal valve   4–6 cm^2
- Mild MS   2–4 cm^2
- Moderate MS   1–2 cm^2
- Severe MS   <1 cm^2.

Criteria for diagnosis of severe MS (many derived from Doppler)

- Measured valve orifice area <1 cm^2
- Mean pressure gradient >10 mmHg
- Pressure half-time >200 ms
- Pulmonary artery systolic pressure >35 mmHg.

A number of diseases produce other typical mitral **M-mode** patterns (Fig. 2.8):

- *LA myxoma.* This has a characteristic appearance. There are multiple echoes filling the space between the MV leaflets. There may initially be an echo-free zone which is filled with echo reflections as the myxoma prolapses through the MV from LA into LV. Other potential causes of a similar echo appearance are large MV vegetations, LA thrombus or aneurysm of the MV.

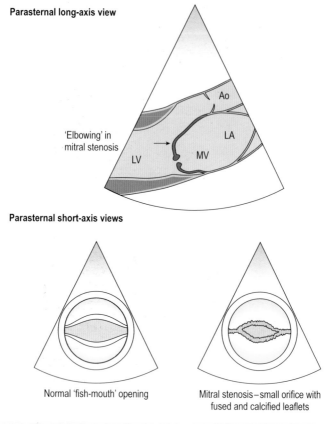

Parasternal long-axis view

Ao

LA

'Elbowing' in mitral stenosis

LV

MV

Parasternal short-axis views

Normal 'fish-mouth' opening

Mitral stenosis – small orifice with fused and calcified leaflets

Fig. 2.6 *2-D echo in mitral stenosis.*

- *Hypertrophic cardiomyopathy (HCM).* In diastole, the valve may be normal, but in systole the entire MV apparatus moves anteriorly producing a characteristic bulge touching the interventricular septum. This is called systolic anterior motion (SAM) of the MV.

- *MV prolapse.* This may be asymptomatic or cause varying degrees of MR. Either anterior or posterior valve leaflets may prolapse into the LA cavity in late systole. This produces an audible click and a late systolic murmur.

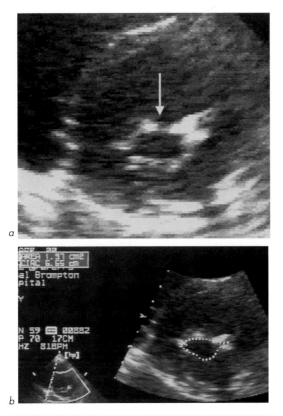

a

b

Fig. 2.7 *Rheumatic mitral stenosis.* **(a)** *Parasternal short-axis view at mitral level showing restricted orifice (arrow) and* **(b)** *valve orifice area calculated by computer software as 1.9 cm².*

- *Flail posterior leaflet.* This may occur as a result of chordal rupture (due to degeneration) or to papillary muscle dysfunction. The posterior leaflet shows erratic movement, rather than the normal 'W' pattern.

- *Aortic regurgitation (AR).* The regurgitant jet passes during diastole along the anterior MV leaflet, causing fluttering vibration of the leaflet and restricting its normal pattern of movement. With increasing severity of AR, the MV is

29

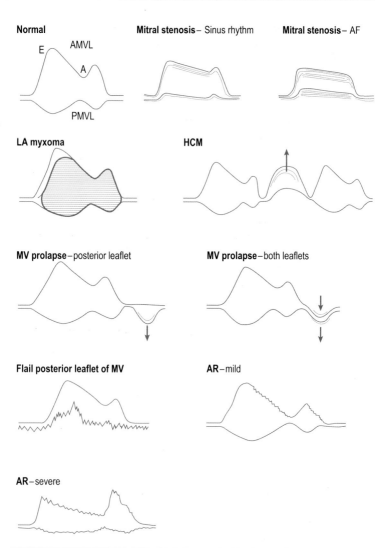

Fig. 2.8 *Mitral valve M-mode patterns.*

more restricted and there may be 'functional' MS (with an anatomically normal MV) giving rise to the diastolic Austin Flint murmur.

Mitral regurgitation (MR)

This is leakage of blood through the MV from LV into LA during ventricular systole. It ranges from very mild to very severe, when the majority of the LV volume empties into the LA rather than into the aorta with each cardiac cycle. A small amount of MR occurs during the closure of many normal MVs – in some series in up to one-third of normal hearts.

In MR, there are changes in:
- The function of the MV
- The LV, which becomes dilated, volume-overloaded and hyperdynamic to maintain cardiac output, since a large proportion of each stroke volume is regurgitating into the LA
- The LA, which becomes dilated.

Echo may show:
- An underlying MV abnormality, e.g. flail MV leaflet with chaotic movement, MV prolapse, vegetations
- Rapid diastolic MV closure due to rapid filling
- Dilated LV with rapid filling (dimensions relate to prognosis)
- Septal and posterior wall motion becomes more vigorous
- Increased circumferential fibre shortening with good LV function
- LA size increased
- Doppler shows size and site of regurgitant jet.

Echo assessment of severity of MR

While the diagnosis of MR may be easy (Fig. 2.9), the echo assessment of severity can be difficult. A balance must be made of all the echo information. The severity relates to the regurgitant fraction, which depends on:
- The size of the regurgitant orifice
- The length of time for which it remains open
- The systolic pressure difference between LV and LA across the valve
- The distensibility of the LA.

Chronic MR

1. Leaflet abnormalities
- rheumatic heart disease – usually in association with mitral stenosis
- MV prolapse ('floppy mitral valve')
- endocarditis
- connective tissue disorders – Marfan's, Ehlers–Danlos, pseudoxanthoma elasticum, osteogenesis imperfecta, SLE
- trauma
- congenital – cleft MV or parachute MV

2. Annulus abnormalities
(circumference usually 10 cm)
- dilatation due to LV dysfunction, e.g. dilated cardiomyopathy or following myocardial infarction. This causes 'functional' MR
- annular calcification – idiopathic, increasing with age, or associated with other conditions, e.g. hypertension, diabetes, aortic stenosis, hypertrophic cardiomyopathy (HCM), hyperparathyroidism, Marfan's

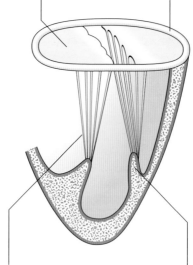

3. Abnormalities of the chordae tendineae
(rupture – more commonly the posterior leaflet)
- idiopathic
- endocarditis
- rheumatic heart disease
- mitral valve prolapse
- Marfan's
- osteogenesis imperfecta

4. Papillary muscle abnormalities
- ischaemia or infarction
- LV dilatation
- rheumatic heart disease
- HCM
- infiltration – sarcoid, amyloid
- myocarditis

Acute MR
- acute myocardial infarction (papillary muscle dysfunction or infarction)
- endocarditis
- chordal rupture

Fig. 2.9 Causes of mitral regurgitation.

The features of severe chronic MR are those of:

1. Volume overload of the LV – dilatation with hyperdynamic movement
2. Volume overload of the LA – dilatation
3. Large regurgitant volume – broad jet extending far into the LA
4. Abnormal valve function.

M-mode shows LV dimensions are increased, as is velocity of motion of the posterior wall and interventricular septum (IVS). The LA is enlarged. There may be features of an underlying cause of MR, e.g. multiple echoes suggesting vegetations due to endocarditis, MV prolapse or flail posterior leaflet.

    2-D echo helps to suggest an underlying cause and assess its consequences. The parasternal long- and short-axis views and apical 4-chamber views are the most helpful and may show:

1. LV abnormality – dilatation causing annular stretching and 'functional' MR, regional wall motion abnormality due to MI or ischaemia, volume-overloaded LV
2. Leaflet abnormalities – rheumatic leaflets, vegetations due to endocarditis, prolapse, flail leaflet
3. Chordae – rupture, thickening, shortening, calcification, vegetations
4. Papillary muscles – rupture, hypertrophy, scarring, calcification.

Doppler echo features of severe MR (Fig. 2.10):

1. Wide jet. The width of the MR jet at the level of the leaflet tips (broad colour flow signal) correlates with severity (a wider jet represents more severe MR).
2. Jet fills a large area of LA. The extent to which the MR jet fills the LA cavity is also an indication. The area of colour in the LA depends on the machine settings and is controversial. However, an area >8 cm^2 is likely to be severe, <4 cm^2 likely to be mild.
3. Systolic flow reversal in pulmonary veins. The jet extends to the pulmonary veins. This can be seen on colour flow mapping and may also cause retrograde flow (LA to lungs) detected by pulsed wave Doppler with the sample volume in one of the pulmonary veins.
4. Dense signal on continuous Doppler. The intensity of the jet is greater with more severe MR since more red cells reflect ultrasound.
5. Raised pulmonary artery (PA) pressure. This is estimated by Doppler from tricuspid regurgitation (TR) (Ch. 3).

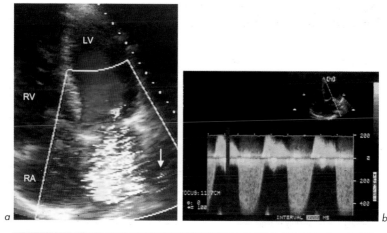

Fig. 2.10 *Severe mitral regurgitation. (a) Colour flow mapping shows a broad jet filling the left atrium and extending into pulmonary veins (arrow). (b) Continuous wave Doppler.*

It is important to know that severe *acute* MR (e.g. due to papillary muscle rupture in acute MI) may not have all these echo features. There is not the time for the features of LV and LA dilatation to develop. A recently occurring narrow high velocity jet of MR into a normal-sized LA may cause a significant rise in LA pressure and symptoms such as breathlessness and signs such as acute pulmonary oedema.

ASE Guidelines to assess severity of mitral regurgitation are shown below.

Mitral valve prolapse (Figs 2.11, 2.12)

This is a common condition affecting up to 5% of the population. There is a wide clinical spectrum. It is also known as floppy or billowing MV. It can cause anything from an audible click to severe MR. It may be an isolated finding or associated with other conditions, such as Marfan's syndrome, secundum ASD, Turner's syndrome, Ehlers–Danlos syndrome or other collagen disorders.

The MV leaflets have increased (redundant) tissue and there may be progressive stretching of these and of the chordae. Individuals often have atypical non-anginal chest pains and palpitations. There is a risk of endocarditis (antibiotic

Severity of mitral regurgitation (MR) – ASE Guidelines

	Mild	Moderate	Severe
Jet area	<4 cm² or <20% LA area	20–40% LA area	>40% LA area
Vena contracta width*	<0.3 cm	0.3–0.7 cm	>0.7 cm
Regurgitant volume	<30 mL	30–59 mL	>60 mL
Regurgitant fraction	<30%	30–49%	>50%
Regurgitant orifice area	<0.2 cm²	0.2–0.39 cm²	>0.4 cm²

*The vena contracta is the narrowest diameter of the jet flow stream that occurs at or just downstream from the orifice. It characteristically has high velocity, laminar flow and is slightly smaller than the anatomical regurgitant orifice due to boundary effects. The cross-sectional area reflects the effective regurgitant orifice area, which is the narrowest area of actual flow. The diameter of the regurgitant orifice is independent of flow rate and driving pressure (for a fixed orifice). It is estimated from colour flow Doppler. Because of the small values of the width of the vena contracta (usually <1 cm), small errors in measurement can lead to a large % error and misjudgement of severity of regurgitation. Hence the importance of accurate acquisition of primary data and measurement.

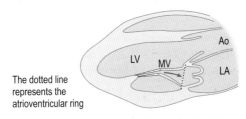

The dotted line represents the atrioventricular ring

Fig. 2.11 *Prolapse of anterior and posterior mitral valve leaflets.*

prophylaxis advice is safest for all dental treatment and surgery) and complications may develop such as progressive MR, embolization, arrhythmias and sudden death.

There are characteristic M-mode and 2-D echo appearances. The echo diagnosis is made if there is systolic movement of part of either MV leaflet above the plane of the annulus in a long-axis view.

2.2 AORTIC VALVE (AV)

The AV is located at the junction of the LV outflow tract and the ascending aorta. The valve usually has 3 cusps (leaflets) – one is located on the anterior wall (right

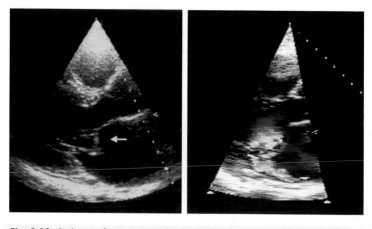

Fig. 2.12 *Prolapse of anterior mitral valve leaflet (arrow) on parasternal long-axis view. This leads to an eccentric jet of mitral regurgitation along the posterior wall of left atrium.*

cusp), and 2 are located on the posterior wall (left and posterior cusps). Behind each cusp, the aortic wall bulges to form an aortic sinus of Valsalva. The coronary arteries arise from the sinuses (right coronary – anterior sinus, left coronary – left posterior sinus) (Fig 2.13).

The AV can be studied by M-mode, 2-D and Doppler techniques. In the parasternal long-axis view, the AV cusps can be seen to open and close on 2-D imaging and an M-mode can be obtained (Figs 1.11b, 2.14).

The aortic cusps form a central closure line in diastole. In systole, the cusps open and close again at end-systole when the aortic pressure exceeds the LV pressure, to form a parallelogram shape. Rarely, echoes from the left coronary cusp may be seen within the parallelogram. The LV ejection time can be measured from the point of cusp opening to cusp closing. It is possible to measure aortic root diameter and LA diameter from this M-mode image.

A number of abnormal patterns of AV movement on M-mode are seen (Fig. 2.15):

- *Bicuspid AV*. This congenital abnormality affects 1–2% of the population and results in cusps which separate normally but usually have an eccentric closure line which may lie anteriorly or posteriorly. (Note that in up to 15% of cases, the closure line is central.) An eccentric closure line may alternatively be

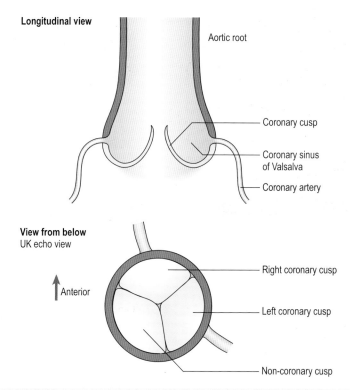

Fig. 2.13 *Aortic valve and root.*

caused in a tricuspid AV when there is a subaortic VSD and prolapse of the right coronary cusp. 2-D echo (especially the parasternal short-axis view at AV level) can help to differentiate between a bicuspid and a tricuspid AV, but this can be difficult if the valve is heavily calcified. Bicuspid AV is an important cause of AS and may co-exist with other congenital abnormalities such as coarctation of the aorta.

- *Calcific AS.* There are dense echoes usually throughout systole and diastole, which may make cusp movement hard to see.
- *Vegetations.* These can usually be seen by echo if 2 mm or more in diameter (transoesophageal echocardiography (TOE) may visualize smaller vegetations (section 5.1)). These usually give multiple echoes in diastole, but if large can

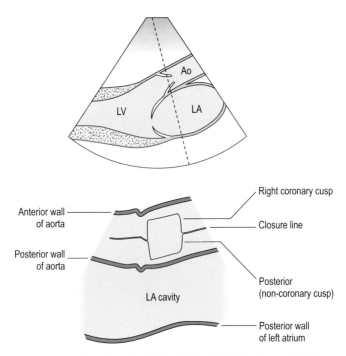

Fig. 2.14 *M-mode at aortic valve and left atrium level.*

also be seen during systole. Distinction from calcific aortic stenosis can be difficult on M-mode.

- *Fibromuscular ring* (*subaortic stenosis*). There is immediate systolic closure of the AV, usually best seen on the right coronary cusp. The valve cusp may not return to its full open position during systole. This is usually best seen on 2-D echo.
- *HCM.* Premature closure of the AV occurs in midsystole due to LVOTO when the IVS and AMVL meet.
- *Prosthetic* (*artificial*) *AV.* Different types of valve produce various appearances, related to the sewing ring, ball or discs (Ch. 6).

Aortic stenosis (AS)

AS may occur at 3 levels – valvular, subvalvular or supravalvular.

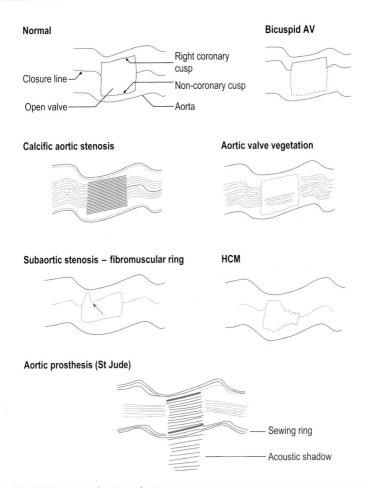

Fig. 2.15 *Aortic valve M-mode patterns.*

Valvular AS. Has 3 main causes:

1. Rheumatic heart disease. Rarely occurs in isolation (2%) and usually in association with mitral disease.

2. Calcific (degenerative) AS associated with increasing age. The commonest cause in Western countries. Minor thickening of AV is found in 20% of those

39

>65 years and 40% of those >75 years. This can progress. Aortic sclerosis is a term that should be avoided as it implies a benign course, which is not always correct.

3. Congenital bicuspid valve (1–2% of population) – a bicuspid AV is found in 40% of middle-aged individuals with AS and 80% of elderly individuals with AS.

Subvalvular AS. Is caused by obstruction proximal to the AV:
1. Subaortic membrane
2. HCM
3. Tunnel subaortic obstruction
4. Upper septal bulge. This is due to fibrosis and hypertrophy, usually in elderly individuals. It unusually may cause obstruction.

Supravalvular AS. This occurs in some congenital conditions such as Williams syndrome (which includes hypercalcaemia, growth failure and mental retardation).

Clinical evidence of severe AS

Echo is an excellent and important method of assessing the degree of severity of AS, but remember there are important **clinical** features which might suggest severe AS.

A mnemonic may help you to remember these features – symptoms and signs – which can be predicted from simple physiology:

Symptoms of severe AS – 5 A's

1. **A**symptomatic – AS is often an incidental finding.
2. **A**ngina – even with normal coronary arteries. Due to increased LV oxygen demand, due to raised wall stress or LVH and supply – demand imbalance.
3. **A**rrhythmia – causing palpitations.
4. **A**ttacks of unconsciousness, i.e. syncope. May be due to arrhythmia or LVOTO but not always related to pressure gradient across the valve.
5. '**A**sthma' (cardiac), i.e. breathlessness, due to raised LV diastolic pressure. Not true asthma. Pulmonary oedema (which can cause bronchospasm and wheezing) due to LV failure in severe AS is a very serious – often fatal – occurrence, taking place late in the disease process.

Signs of severe AS – 4 S's

1. **S**low-rising pulse – due to LVOTO.
2. **S**ystolic blood pressure low – due to LVOTO.
3. **S**ustained apex beat – due to LVH from pressure overload. The apex is not displaced as the external heart size does not increase – the heart hypertrophies 'inwards'.
4. **S**econd heart sound abnormalities – these range from soft, narrow-split, single (only P_2 heard), reversed split (A_2–P_2 splitting paradoxically shorter in inspiration) based on severity of AS, effect upon LV ejection time and mobility of aortic cusps.

One very important fact to remember: The severity of AS is **NOT** related to the loudness of the murmur. Turbulent flow across a mildly narrowed valve can cause a very loud murmur. Conversely, a very severely narrowed valve may cause marked restriction to blood flow and may be associated with only a very soft murmur.

Echo features of AS

The **M-mode** features of AS have been mentioned. On **2-D echo** using parasternal long- and short-axis views and apical 5-chamber views:

1. The cusps may be seen to be thickened, calcified, have reduced motion or may 'dome' (the latter is usually diagnostic of AS).
2. There may be LVH due to pressure overload.
3. LV dilatation occurs if heart failure has developed (usually a poor prognostic feature).
4. Post-stenotic dilatation of the aorta may be seen.

Doppler is most useful in determining the severity of AS by estimating the pressure gradient across the AV (Fig. 2.16). Valve area can be calculated by use of the continuity equation (Ch. 3).

Severity of AS correlates with valve area, peak velocity, peak pressure gradient and mean pressure gradient (often more accurate than peak).

The AV pressure gradients depend on cardiac output. They can be overestimated in high-output states (e.g. anaemia) and underestimated in low-output states (e.g. systolic heart failure). The continuity equation helps in this case (Fig. 3.13).

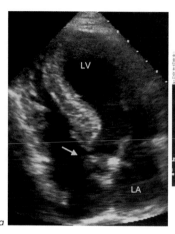
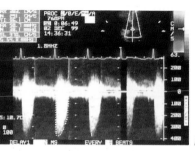

Fig. 2.16 *Calcific aortic stenosis.* **(a)** *The calcified aortic valve is shown (arrow) in this apical 5-chamber view.* **(b)** *Continuous Doppler shows a peak velocity of 3.7 m/s (peak gradient of 54 mmHg).*

Features of varying degrees of AS		
	Valve area (cm²)	
Normal	2.5–3.5	
Mild	1.5–2.5	
Moderate	0.75–1.5	
Severe	<0.75	
	Peak velocity (m/s)	**Peak gradient (mmHg)**	**Mean gradient (mmHg)**
Normal	1.0	<10	<10
Mild	1.0–2.0	<20	<20
Moderate	2.0–4.0	20–64	20–40
Severe	>4.0	>64	>40

Surgical intervention (valve replacement)

This is indicated in:

- Severe AS (maximum gradient >64 mmHg, mean gradient >40 mmHg)
- AS of lesser extent with symptoms (e.g. syncope)

- Severe AS with LV systolic dysfunction
- Severe/moderate AS at other cardiac surgery (e.g. coronary bypass)
- Asymptomatic severe AS with expected high exertion or pregnancy.

Aortic regurgitation (AR) (Fig. 2.17)

This is leakage of blood from the aorta into the LV during diastole.

Echo diagnosis of AR

All the echo modalities are useful in diagnosis and evaluation. Doppler and colour flow mapping are especially helpful. M-mode and 2-D echo cannot directly diagnose AR but may indicate underlying causes (e.g. dilated aortic root, bicuspid AV) and aid in the assessment of the effects of AR (e.g. LV dilatation).

M-mode may show:

- Vegetations on AV
- Fluttering of AV cusps in diastole (e.g. rupture due to endocarditis or degeneration)

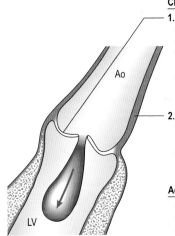

Chronic AR

1. Valvular
- endocarditis
- rheumatic heart disease
- congenital – bicuspid valve, subaortic and supraaortic stenosis
- connective tissue and inflammatory disease – rheumatoid arthritis, SLE, Crohn's, ankylosing spondylitis, Whipple's

2. Aortic root diseases
- dilatation – Marfan's, hypertension, Ehlers–Danlos, pseudoxanthoma elasticum, aortitis
- distortion – dissection (types I and II), syphilis, ankylosing spondylitis, Reiter's, rupture of sinus of Valsalva aneurysm

Acute AR
- endocarditis
- dissection
- trauma

Fig. 2.17 *Causes of aortic regurgitation.*

43

- Eccentric closure line of bicuspid valve
- Dilatation of aortic root
- Fluttering of anterior MV leaflet
- Premature opening of AV because of raised left ventricular end-diastolic pressure (LVEDP) and premature closure of MV. Both suggest severe AR
- Dilatation of LV cavity due to volume overload
- Exaggerated septal and posterior wall of LV wall motion (exaggerated septal early dip strongly suggests AR).

2-D echo may show:

- LV dilatation – correlates with severity of AR
- Abnormal leaflets (bicuspid, rheumatic)
- Vegetations
- Dilated aortic root
- Proximal aortic dissection
- Abnormal indentation of the anterior MV leaflet
- Abnormal intraventricular septal motion.

Doppler

This is useful both for detecting AR and assessing its severity. Colour flow mapping is helpful. The jet of AR can be seen entering the LV cavity on a number of views such as parasternal long axis and apical 5-chamber. Pulsed Doppler can be used in the apical 5-chamber view with the sample volume just proximal to the AV. AR can be detected as a signal above the baseline (towards the transducer) but since AR velocity is usually high (>2 m/s) aliasing will occur. Continuous wave Doppler is then useful and the signal seen only above the baseline (Fig. 2.18).

There are 2 possible complicating factors:

1. The AR jet may be missed, especially if eccentric. Colour flow mapping can detect the jet and aid in placing the pulse wave sample volume, which can be moved around the entire LV outflow tract in a number of different views.
2. The AR jet may be difficult to differentiate from a high-velocity jet of MS, especially in 5–chamber view (the 2 often co-exist!).

Colour flow can confirm which or if both conditions are present and pulsed Doppler is used to map the LV outflow tract and MV areas separately. Continuous

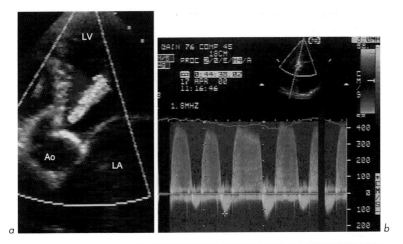

Fig. 2.18 *Mild aortic regurgitation. (a) Zoomed apical 5-chamber view showing a narrow jet extending a short distance into LV cavity on colour flow mapping. (b) Continuous wave Doppler. Note beat-to-beat variation since subject is in atrial fibrillation.*

Doppler of AR shows a velocity signal starting early in and lasting throughout diastole with a high peak velocity (>2 m/s). MS produces a mid-diastolic velocity signal, usually with a peak velocity of <2 m/s.

Assessing the severity of AR

As with MR, assessing severity of AR is not straightforward. A number of echo criteria are used:

1. Effects on the LV
2. The volume of blood regurgitating across the valve
3. The rate of fall of the pressure gradient between the aorta and LV.

M-mode and 2-D echo show LV dilatation with severe AR. Progressive dilatation with symptoms or left ventricular end-systolic diameter (LVESD) in excess of 5.5 cm are indications for surgical intervention.

Doppler is quite good at indicating severe AR (Fig. 2.19) but not so good at distinguishing between mild and moderate AR.

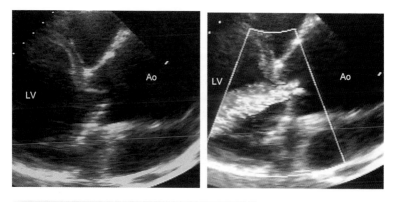

Fig. 2.19 *Severe aortic regurgitation due to aneurysmal dilatation of aortic root. Parasternal long-axis views.*

Using **pulsed wave Doppler**, the sample volume can be placed in various positions within the LV cavity to give a semi-quantitative idea of severity by seeing how far into the LV cavity the AR jet reaches. As a broad rule of thumb, mild AR remains within the area of the AV, moderate AR remains between the left ventricular outflow tract (LVOT) and the level of the MV above papillary muscle level and severe AR extends to the LV apex.

This only gives a rough approximation – a narrow jet of mild AR may extend deep into the LV cavity, while a severe broad jet of AR may be eccentrically angled and not extend far into the LV.

Using **colour flow mapping**, the width of the AR jet immediately below the AV indicates severity. This relates to the area of failed valvular apposition (the regurgitant orifice). A jet width >60% of aortic width at cusp level is usually severe. A frozen image of AR can be taken and planimetry used to estimate the cross-sectional area of the jet. The length of the AR jet into the LV cavity on apical 5-chamber view can also indicate severity (longer jet – more severe AR).

With **continuous wave Doppler**, the slope of the deceleration rate of the Doppler signal of AR can give an indication of severity as can the intensity of the signal (more intense – more severe AR). The basis for this is described in Chapter 3. Diastolic flow reversal in the aortic arch also suggests severe AR.

As with acute-onset MR, these echo features of severe AR may not all be present in *acute* AR (e.g. due to endocarditis which has destroyed the valve, dissection of the ascending aorta or trauma). The LV cavity has not had time to dilate and so even a relatively small-volume high-velocity jet of AR into the LV may cause a rise in LVEDP which causes breathlessness and may cause pulmonary oedema.

ASE Guidelines to assess severity of aortic regurgitation are shown below.

Severity of aortic regurgitation (AR) – ASE Guidelines			
	Mild	**Moderate**	**Severe**
Jet width/LVOT	<25%	25–64%	>65%
Vena contracta width*	<0.3 cm	0.3–0.6 cm	>0.6 cm
Jet density continuous wave Doppler	Incomplete or faint	Dense	Dense
Pressure half-time	Slow >500 ms	Medium 200–500 ms	Steep <200 ms
Regurgitant volume	<30 mL	30–59 mL	>60 mL
Regurgitant volume	<30 mL/beat	30–59 mL/beat	>60 mL/beat
Regurgitant fraction	<30%	30–49%	>50%
Regurgitant orifice area	<0.1 cm^2	0.1–0.29 cm^2	>0.3 cm^2

*The vena contracta is the narrowest diameter of the flow stream. It reflects the diameter of the regurgitant orifice and is independent of flow rate and driving pressure.

Indications for surgery in AR

The timing of surgical repair of chronic AR is a difficult decision. Progressive LV dilatation and/or impairment can indicate the need for valve replacement. This is particularly true if symptoms develop (e.g. breathlessness, reduced exercise capacity). The main indications are:

- Symptomatic severe AR with or without LV systolic dysfunction
- Asymptomatic severe AR with LV systolic dysfunction or dilatation, particularly if progressive (ejection fraction <50%, LVESD >55 mm).

In acute AR, urgent surgery is often based clinically upon the degree of haemodynamic compromise and the underlying cause (e.g. dissection of the aorta).

2.3 TRICUSPID VALVE (TV)

Tricuspid stenosis (TS)

Abnormalities of the TV should not be overlooked. It is not unknown for rheumatic MS to be surgically repaired, only for it to be subsequently discovered that the diagnosis of co-existent rheumatic TS was not made preoperatively!

The TV is structurally similar to the MV in having:

* Leaflets – the TV has 3, as its name suggests, unlike the 2 of the MV
* Chordae attached to papillary muscles (subvalvular apparatus)
* An annulus or valve ring – which has a larger area than that of the MV, normal TV area 5–8 cm^2.

The most common cause of TS is rheumatic heart disease. There is nearly always co-existent MS. TS occurs about 10 times less commonly. Other rare causes of TS include carcinoid syndrome (excessive secretion of 5-hydroxytryptamine (5-HT) usually from a malignant intra-abdominal tumour causes TS, asthma, flushing etc.; often associated with TR); right atrium (RA) tumours (e.g. myxoma causing obstruction); obstruction of RV inflow tract (rare – vegetations, extracardiac tumours, pericardial constriction); congenital (Ebstein's anomaly, Ch. 6) or right-sided endocarditis (intravenous drug abusers or following cannulation of veins).

M-mode and 2-D echo findings are analogous to MS:

* Thick and/or calcified leaflets
* Restricted leaflet motion
* Doming of one or more leaflets in diastole (especially the anterior leaflet).

In rheumatic disease, the leaflets are thick and the tips are fused. In carcinoid, the tips tend to be separate and mobile.

Doppler findings are similar to MS. Trans-tricuspid flow is best measured with pulsed Doppler in the apical 4-chamber view with the sample volume in the RV immediately below the TV. There is increased flow velocity in diastole. Evaluation of severity is rarely needed in clinical practice, but is by similar principles as indicated for MS (diastolic pressure gradient and valve area). Severe TS is usually associated with a gradient of 3–10 mmHg.

The pressure half-time equation used for MS (Ch. 3) is empirical and the constant should not be applied to TS.

Tricuspid regurgitation (TR) (Figs 2.20, 2.21)

Virtually every TV shows some TR during its normal function. This fact allows the use of Doppler echo to estimate PASP (Ch. 3).

Causes of TR are similar to MR – the commonest causes are secondary to RV dilatation (dilating the TV annulus), and primary causes include disease of the leaflets, and/or the subvalvular apparatus.

Secondary causes – most common

- PHT
- Pulmonary valve disease
- Cor pulmonale (right heart failure associated with lung disease such as emphysema)
- Ischaemic heart disease
- Cardiomyopathies
- Volume overload (e.g. ASD, VSD)
- Interference with normal valve closure (e.g. pacing lead).

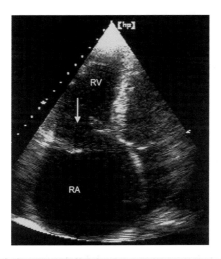

Fig. 2.20 Prolapse of the tricuspid valve (apical 4-chamber view).

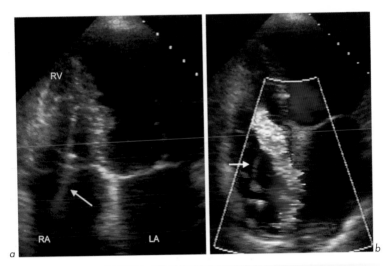

Fig. 2.21 *Pacing wire.* **(a)** *The wire (arrow) passes through the tricuspid valve from right atrium to right ventricle.* **(b)** *Associated with an eccentric jet of tricuspid regurgitation. Apical 4-chamber views.*

Primary causes

- Infective endocarditis
- Rheumatic heart disease
- Carcinoid
- Chordal rupture
- Papillary muscle dysfunction
- TV prolapse
- Connective tissue diseases
- Rheumatoid arthritis
- Congenital, e.g. Ebstein's anomaly.

Echo assessment of TR severity is best achieved by Doppler as with MR. More severe TR is associated with a broad, high-intensity jet filling the RA. There is associated retrograde systolic flow in the vena cava and hepatic vein.

2.4 PULMONARY VALVE (PV)

The PV has 3 leaflets and sits at the junction of the RV outflow tract (RVOT) and the main pulmonary artery (PA).

Pulmonary stenosis (PS)

As with AS, PS may be valvular, supravalvular (peripheral) or subvalvular (infundibular).

Valvular PS may be congenital (most common – isolated, or as part of another syndrome, e.g. Noonan's, tetralogy of Fallot or rubella) or acquired (rheumatic, carcinoid).

Assessment of severity is along similar principles to AS. **2-D echo** may show thickened, calcified leaflets, doming of the valve leaflets in systole and restricted motion. There may be post-stenotic dilatation of the PA or its branches and RV hypertrophy or dilatation due to pressure overload.

The normal peak velocity across the valve is 1.0 m/s. The peak gradient across the valve can be estimated by **Doppler**. This correlates with estimated valve area.

Severity of PS	Peak gradient (mmHg)	Valve area (cm²)
Mild	<25	>1.0
Moderate	25–40	0.5–1.0
Severe	>40	<0.5

There may be few symptoms and quite severe PS may be well tolerated into adult life.

Supravalvular PS can be due to stenosis of the main PA or any of its branches distal to the PV (e.g. rubella – often with PDA or infantile hypercalcaemia – with supraaortic stenosis). It may be iatrogenic – post-surgical banding of the PA which is performed in some left to right shunts as a temporary measure to protect the pulmonary circulation.

One or more discrete shelf-like bands may be seen in the PA on 2-D echo. A long stenotic tapering tunnel area may be seen distal to the PV. The increase in Doppler velocity detected by pulsed wave Doppler is distal to and not at the level of the PV.

Subvalvular PS is most commonly congenital – rarely isolated, usually in association with valvular stenosis, VSD, tetralogy of Fallot and transposition of the great arteries. May also occur in hypertrophic cardiomyopathies. Acquired causes, e.g. tumours, are very rare.

A muscular band and/or narrowing of the subvalvular area are seen. There is not usually post-stenotic dilatation. Using pulsed wave Doppler, it can be seen that the increase in velocity occurs in the RVOT below the level of the PV.

Pulmonary regurgitation (PR)

Secondary causes – most common
- Dilatation of the PA – PHT, Marfan's.

Primary causes
- Infective endocarditis
- Rheumatic heart disease
- Carcinoid
- Congenital (e.g. absence or malformation of PV leaflets, or following surgery for tetralogy of Fallot)
- Iatrogenic (e.g. post-valvotomy or catheter-induced at angiography)
- Syphilis.

M-mode and 2-D echo cannot detect PR directly but can show some evidence of the underlying cause and the effect. There may be evidence of:
- PHT – dilated RV, dilated PA, abnormal IVS motion (behaves as though it 'belongs' to the RV rather than LV – 'right ventricularization' of IVS)
- Dilated PA – the diameter can be measured usually in parasternal short-axis view at AV level
- Vegetation on the valve in endocarditis
- Thick immobile PV leaflets in rheumatic heart disease or carcinoid
- Absent valve leaflets (congenital)
- PA aneurysm.

Doppler techniques show PR and help to assess severity, as with AR. Doppler indicators of severe PR are:

- Colour flow – the regurgitant jet is visualized directly. Severity is indicated by the width of the jet at valve level, how far into RV it extends and the area of the jet by planimetry.
- Pulsed wave Doppler – the distance between the PV and the level at which PR is detected can be determined. A jet at the lower infundibular region is severe.
- Increased intensity of the Doppler signal.
- Increased slope of the Doppler signal (deceleration time).

CHAPTER 3

Doppler – velocities and pressures

3.1 SPECIAL USES OF DOPPLER

The Doppler effect (Fig. 3.1), described by the Austrian physicist and mathematician Christian Johann Doppler in 1842, is a change in the frequency of sound, light or other waves caused by the motion of the source or the observer. An example is the change in the sound of an ambulance siren as it approaches (higher pitch) and then passes (lower pitch) an observer. The change is due to compression and rarefaction of sound waves. There is a direct relationship between the relative velocity of the sound source and the observer and the change in pitch.

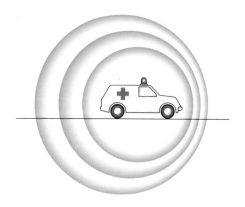

Fig. 3.1 *Doppler effect.*

Measuring blood velocity and pressure gradients

The Doppler effect can be used to examine the direction and velocity of blood flow in blood vessels and within the heart. Ultrasound waves of a known frequency (usually around 2 MHz) are transmitted from the transducer and are reflected by moving blood back towards the transducer, which also acts as an ultrasound receiver. If the blood is moving towards the transducer, the frequency of the ultrasound signal increases and vice versa. This can be used by computer analysis to derive haemodynamic information such as the nature and severity of valvular abnormalities (e.g. valvular stenosis) since it is possible to relate velocity to pressure difference (also referred to as pressure gradient) by a simple equation (below). Doppler can also detect the presence of valvular regurgitation and give an indication of its severity. This information can complement the anatomical information provided by M-mode and 2-D echo techniques. The Doppler-measured flow patterns and velocities across the heart valves can be displayed graphically against time on the screen of the echo machine or printed on paper. By convention, velocities towards the transducer are displayed above the line and those away from it below the line. The normal flow patterns for the aortic and mitral valves are shown below (Figs 3.2 and 3.3).

This is a graph of velocity against time, but it also gives a densitometric dimension, since the density of any spot is related to the strength of the reflected signal, which relates to the number of reflecting red blood cells moving at that velocity. In normal situations where blood flow is laminar (smooth), most of the blood cells travel at more-or-less the same velocity, accelerating and decelerating

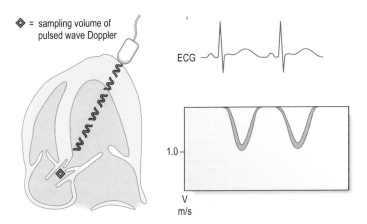

Fig. 3.2 *Normal laminar flow across aortic valve.*

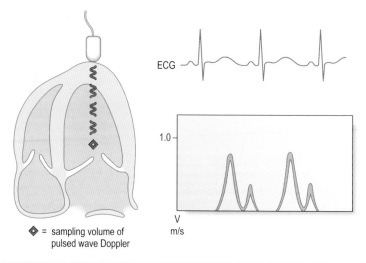

Fig. 3.3 *Normal laminar flow across mitral valve.*

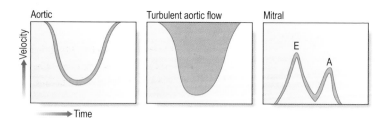

Fig. 3.4 *Normal laminar pulsed wave Doppler patterns and turbulent aortic flow pattern.*

together (Fig. 3.4). The Doppler pattern then has an outline form with very few cells travelling at other velocities at a given time. When there is turbulence of flow, e.g. due to a narrowed valve, there is a wide distribution of blood cell velocities, and the Doppler signal is 'filled in'.

Note that for aortic flow the blood is moving away from the transducer placed at the cardiac apex and the Doppler signal is displayed below the baseline. The opposite is true for mitral flow which is predominantly towards the apex.

The peak Doppler velocities in normal adults and children are (in m/s):

Valve	Peak	Range
Aortic valve/aorta	1.3	(0.9–1.7)
Left ventricle	0.9	(0.7–1.1)
Mitral valve	0.9	(0.6–1.3)
Tricuspid valve	0.5	(0.3–0.7)
Pulmonary valve/artery	0.75	(0.5–1.0)

Doppler can be used to measure velocities and estimate pressure gradients across narrowed (stenosed) valves.

The normal stroke volume in a resting adult is approximately 70 mL. This volume of blood passes across the AV with each ventricular systole, at a blood velocity of approximately 1 m/s. If the AV is stenosed, with a smaller valve orifice cross-sectional area, then for the same volume of blood to be ejected, the blood must accelerate, and this increase in velocity can be measured using Doppler with the ultrasound transducer at the cardiac apex and transmitting sound waves continuously (Fig. 3.5). Since the blood is moving away from the echo transducer, the Doppler velocity signal is below the baseline. In this case, the peak blood velocity across the AV is 5 m/s.

There is a direct and simple relationship between the velocity of blood across a narrowing (stenosis) and the pressure gradient (drop) across the narrowing (not the absolute pressure). This is known as the simplified *Bernoulli equation*:

$$\Delta P = 4\,V^2$$

where ΔP is the pressure gradient (in mmHg) and V is the peak blood velocity (in m/s) measured by Doppler across the narrowing. In the example shown of AS (Fig. 3.5), the peak Doppler velocity is 5 m/s, which gives an estimated AV gradient of 100 mmHg (severe AS).

Uses and limitations of Doppler

The main advantage of Doppler is that it allows accurate haemodynamic measurements to be made noninvasively. The pressure gradient measured has the added advantage of being a true physiological instantaneous gradient (i.e. a gradient that exists in real-time) unlike the peak-to-peak pressure gradient that

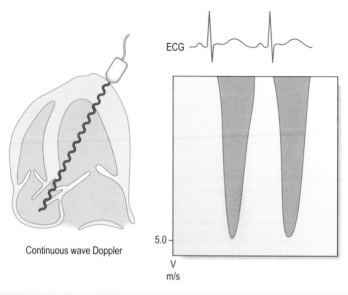

ECG

5.0

V
m/s

Continuous wave Doppler

Fig. 3.5 *Doppler – aortic stenosis.*

is calculated from most cardiac catheterization studies, since the peak LV pressure and peak aortic pressure do not occur simultaneously (Fig. 3.6).

An equation has been derived which approximately relates peak-to-peak aortic pressure gradient (from catheterization) to peak instantaneous Doppler gradient:

$$\text{Peak-to-peak gradient} \simeq (0.84 \times \text{peak Doppler gradient}) - 14\,\text{mmHg}$$

The main limitation of using the Doppler technique is that blood velocity is a vector (it has direction). It is therefore essential that the ultrasound beam is lined up in parallel with the direction of blood flow, otherwise the peak velocity (and consequently the valve pressure gradient) will be underestimated. This can be especially difficult when the direction of the blood flow jet is eccentric due to the anatomy of the stenosed valve (Fig. 3.7).

Another limitation with pulsed wave Doppler is that blood of velocity less than 2 m/s only can be examined. Beyond that an effect known as aliasing occurs and continuous Doppler must be used.

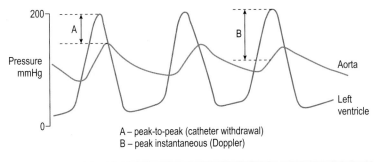

Fig. 3.6 *Doppler measures instantaneous pressure gradient.*

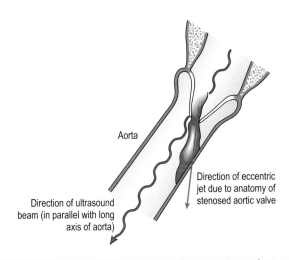

Fig. 3.7 *Continuous wave Doppler may underestimate the velocity of an eccentric jet.*

Mitral stenosis (Fig. 3.8)

The velocity of blood across the healthy MV is approximately 0.9 m/s. In the presence of MS, blood velocity across the valve increases. This can be measured by continuous wave Doppler and an assessment made of severity of valve stenosis and of valve area.

59

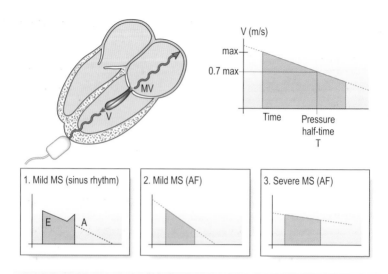

Fig. 3.8 *Mitral stenosis – Doppler assessment of valve area.*

This is done by looking at the way the pressure across the MV varies with time as blood flows across it. If blood flows across a normal valve, there would be a rapid peak of high-velocity blood and the velocity then falls away quickly as the pressures between LA and LV equalize. In a stenosed valve, the peak in velocity is higher, but the time taken for the pressure gradient to fall away is prolonged, and the more severe the stenosis the more slowly the pressure falls away (remember to think of it as the pressure gradient being maintained for a longer period to push blood across a narrowed valve).

It has been found that the area of the mitral valve (A_{MV}) and the time taken for the pressure gradient to fall away to half its initial peak value (T) are approximately inversely proportional to each other.

If A_{MV} is measured in cm^2 and T in milliseconds, the constant has been found empirically to be equal to 220:

$$A_{MV} = \frac{220}{T}$$

So to estimate A_{MV}, it is sufficient to measure T. Doppler does not measure pressure gradient directly, but measures velocity; pressure gradient is derived from the simplified Bernoulli equation. That means that the pressure gradient will have fallen to half its peak value when the velocity has fallen to $1/\sqrt{2}$ of its peak value, i.e. to 0.7 of its peak value.

Measurement of the time T taken for peak blood velocity to reach 0.7 of its value (equivalent to pressure gradient reaching half its value) is called the **pressure half-time** and a good approximation of A_{MV} is:

$$A_{MV} = \frac{220}{\text{Pressure half-time}}$$

Many echo machines have software packages which allow measurement of pressure half-time and estimation of MV area. It is less accurate for very low pressure half-time.

In many cases of severe MS, the rhythm is atrial fibrillation (AF) and there is no second A-wave peak of velocity of the transmitral flow (which is caused by atrial contraction). In this situation, the slope of the top of the Doppler velocity signal can be measured to calculate MV area. Since the heart rate and the duration of systole and diastole vary from beat to beat in AF, it is ideal to measure a number of beats to take the average value of MV area. When the rhythm is normal sinus rhythm, the slope of the top of the early phase of transmitral flow (E-wave) is taken, and the A-wave ignored.

The technique should not be used in determining the severity of tricuspid stenosis as the constant is not the same.

Severity of aortic regurgitation by continuous Doppler

As described in section 2.2, the slope and intensity of the continuous Doppler signal of AR can indicate severity (Fig. 3.9). The greater the slope, the more severe the AR. A steep slope indicates that, as diastole progresses, the pressure gradient across the AV in diastole between the aorta and LV cavity is becoming smaller. The AV is acting less effectively in keeping the 2 areas separated.

Another way to express this is the time taken for the maximum pressure gradient across the AV to drop to half its value – the pressure half-time. The more quickly the pressure difference falls away (or the shorter the pressure half-time), the more severe is the AR (Fig. 3.10).

A correlation has been made between severity and these measurements:

Severity of AR	Deceleration rate of AR (m/s^2)	Pressure half-time (ms)
Mild	<2	>500
Moderate	2–3	200–500
Severe	>3	<200

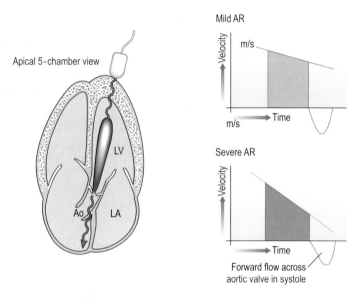

Fig. 3.9 Doppler assessment of severity of aortic regurgitation.

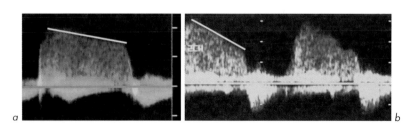

Fig. 3.10 Aortic regurgitation. Continuous Doppler patterns showing **(a)** mild AR and **(b)** severe aortic regurgitation.

The intensity of the continuous wave Doppler signal also gives a qualitative indication of AR severity. It is more intense in severe AR as a greater volume of blood is moving with a given velocity and reflecting ultrasound to the transducer.

PA systolic pressure from tricuspid regurgitation

Doppler can be used to give a noninvasive measurement of pulmonary artery systolic pressure (PASP) (Fig. 3.11).

This technique takes advantage of the fact that a small degree of TR is found in virtually all normal hearts. The pressure gradient which can be measured using the Bernoulli equation is applied to TR to estimate PASP.

This is how it is done:

1. The aim is to measure PASP. Assuming no PV stenosis, then this is equal to right ventricular systolic pressure (RVSP).

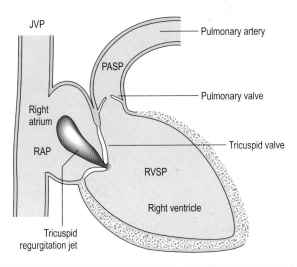

Fig. 3.11 *Doppler estimation of pulmonary artery systolic pressure from velocity of tricuspid regurgitation.*

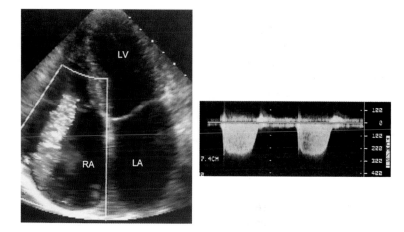

Fig. 3.12 *Tricuspid regurgitation. A broad jet extending far into the right atrium on colour flow mapping. Continuous Doppler shows a peak velocity of 3.1 m/s, giving an estimated pulmonary artery systolic pressure of 39 mmHg + jugular venous pressure.*

2. RVSP can be easily estimated from the maximum velocity of the TR jet (V_{TR}) (Fig. 3.12). The pressure gradient between the right atrium and the right ventricle across the tricuspid valve (RVSP – RAP) can be estimated by the Bernoulli equation using the maximum V_{TR}:

$$RVSP - RAP = 4V_{TR}^2$$

3. The value of RAP is known – it is equal to the jugular venous pressure (JVP) which can be assessed clinically (in healthy individuals and is usually 0–5 cm of blood, measured from the sternal angle, and 1 cm of blood is almost equal to 1 mmHg).

4. This allows us to estimate that:

$$PASP = RVSP = 4V_{TR}^2 + JVP$$

If the measured V_{TR} is 2 m/s and the JVP is 0, this gives an approximate PASP of 16 mmHg. The normal value of PASP is up to 25 mmHg.

Continuity equation

In some situations, the Doppler-estimated peak velocity (and hence pressure gradient) across a valve is not a true indication of the severity of valvular stenosis. An example is AS in the presence of LV systolic impairment. This may arise either as a result of long-standing AS which has caused LV impairment, or of AS co-existing with LV disease, e.g. dilated cardiomyopathy or ischaemic heart failure. In this situation, the impaired LV may not be able to generate a high velocity across the AV.

The severity of AS can be assessed by calculating the AV orifice area using the *continuity equation* (Fig. 3.13), the principle of which is simple – the volume of blood that leaves the LV in a given time must be the same volume that crosses the AV and enters the aorta.

If a cross-sectional area (A) at a level in the LV is calculated (in cm^2, by using M-mode or 2-D measurements) and the velocity of blood (V) at that level measured (in cm/s by using pulsed wave Doppler), the product of area by velocity gives the volume of blood flow at that level in cm^3/s. As explained above, this volume is the same as that crossing the AV and entering the aorta.

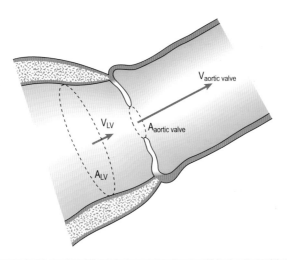

Fig. 3.13 *Continuity equation.*

Use of this can be made to measure the area of interest, at AV level ($A_{aortic\ valve}$). The peak velocity across the aortic valve ($V_{aortic\ valve}$) can also be measured by Doppler:

$$A_{aortic\ valve} \times V_{aortic\ valve} = A_{LV} \times V_{LV}$$

$$A_{aortic\ valve} = \frac{A_{LV} \times V_{LV}}{V_{aortic\ valve}}$$

This is not helpful in AS if the peak velocity is <2 m/s.

CHAPTER 4
Heart failure, myocardium and pericardium

4.1 HEART FAILURE

There is no ideal definition of heart failure. One definition is of a clinical syndrome caused by an abnormality of the heart which leads to a characteristic pattern of haemodynamic, renal, neural and hormonal responses. A shorter definition is ventricular dysfunction with symptoms.

Echo plays a crucial role when heart failure is suspected (e.g. unexplained breathlessness, clinical signs such as raised venous pressure, basal crackles, third heart sound) to help establish the diagnosis, assess ventricular function and institute correct treatment.

An underlying *cause* of heart failure should always be sought and echo plays an essential role here also. The most common cause in Western populations is coronary artery disease. Echo may also reveal a surgically treatable underlying cause, e.g. valvular disease or LV aneurysm. Heart failure may be caused by severe AS (which affects 3% of those aged over 75 years) and the murmur at this stage may be absent.

Major therapeutic advances have been made in the past two decades, including the use of modern diuretics, angiotensin-converting enzyme (ACE) inhibitors, device therapy and cardiac transplantation. This has improved the quality and duration of life of many with heart failure.

Some studies (e.g. Framingham study) have provided epidemiological data on heart failure:

- Incidence is 0.5–1.5% per year, increasing in many countries, because the population is ageing and there has been a reduction in the fatality rate for acute MI
- Almost 50% of patients surviving MI develop heart failure
- Prevalence is 1–3% (above the age of 70 years, it is 5–10%).

The term dilated cardiomyopathy describes large hearts with reduced contractile function in the presence of normal coronary arteries (section 4.4). It is usually of unknown cause. When a cause is established, the term is sometimes preceded by a qualifier, such as alcoholic dilated cardiomyopathy. Hypertension has become a less common cause of heart failure as a consequence of its improved detection and treatment. It remains an important contributory factor to the progression of heart failure and is a risk factor for coronary artery disease.

Causes of chronic heart failure

Myocardial disease
Systolic failure
- Coronary artery disease — Dyskinesia, diffuse dysfunction, aneurysm, incoordination, stunning, hibernation
- Cardiomyopathy — Idiopathic – dilated, hypertrophic, restrictive
  Poisons – alcohol, heavy metals, toxins, poisons, doxorubicin, other cardiotoxic drugs
  Myocarditis
  Endocrine (e.g. hypothyroidism)
  Infiltration – amyloid, endomyocardial fibrosis
- Hypertension
- Drugs — β-blockers, calcium antagonists, antiarrhythmic drugs

Diastolic failure
- Elderly, ischaemia, hypertrophy

Arrhythmias
- Tachycardia — AF, VT, supraventricular tachycardia (SVT)
- Bradycardia — Complete heart block

Pericardial diseases
Valve dysfunction
- Pressure overload — Aortic stenosis
- Volume overload — Mitral or aortic regurgitation
- Restricted forward flow — Mitral or aortic stenosis

Shunts
Extracardiac disease
'High output' failure — Anaemia, thyrotoxicosis, pregnancy, glomerulonephritis, AV fistula, Paget's disease of bone, beri-beri

Adapted from Kaddoura & Poole-Wilson, 1999, *Cardiology,* McGraw-Hill, pp. 523–533.

It is always important to seek the cause of worsening features (decompensation) of heart failure in a previously clinically stable individual. This may lead to symptoms such as breathlessness or signs such as crackles in the chest, raised venous pressure or peripheral oedema. Echo can help in the investigation of the potential causes:

- Non-compliance with medications, e.g. diuretics
- Myocardial infarction or ischaemia
- Cardiac rhythm change, e.g. AF, VT
- Valvular heart disease, e.g. worsening AS or MR
- Progression of myocardial disease, e.g. dilated cardiomyopathy
- Drugs, e.g. β-blockers or other negative inotropes or negative chronotropes
- Infection, e.g. pneumonia, urinary tract infection, cellulitis, endocarditis
- Noncardiac medical conditions, e.g. anaemia, thyroid dysfunction, infection
- Pulmonary disease (e.g. PHT or PE).

There are many causes of *acute* heart failure, the most common of which is myocardial ischaemia or infarction.

Causes of acute heart failure and cardiogenic shock

- Acute MI – extensive LV myocardial damage, acute VSD, acute MR, RV infarction, cardiac rupture
- Decompensation of chronic heart failure – poor compliance with medication, intercurrent illness or infection, arrhythmia (e.g. AF or VT), myocardial ischaemia, anaemia, thyroid disease
- Arrhythmia – tachycardia (e.g. AF, VT or SVT) or bradycardia (e.g. complete heart block)
- Obstruction to cardiac output – critical aortic or mitral stenosis, HOCM, myxoma
- Valvular regurgitation – acute mitral or aortic regurgitation
- Myocarditis
- Acute massive pulmonary embolism
- Myocardial dysfunction following cardiac surgery
- Fluid overload
- Cardiac tamponade
- Cor pulmonale
- Poisoning or drug overdose
- Accelerated hypertension
- Cardiac trauma
- Rejection of heart transplant
- 'High output' heart failure (see 'Causes of chronic heart failure' table)

Adapted from Holmberg, 1996, in *Diseases of the Heart*, Saunders, pp. 456–466 and Dob, 2003, in *Oh's Intensive Care Manual*, Butterworth-Heinemann.

4.2 ASSESSMENT OF LV SYSTOLIC FUNCTION

This is one of the most important and common uses of echo. LV systolic function is a major prognostic factor in cardiac disease and has important implications for treatment. Clinical management is altered if an abnormality is detected (e.g. the diagnosis of systolic heart failure should lead to the initiation of ACE inhibitors unless there is a contraindication).

LV systolic function can be assessed by M-mode, 2-D and Doppler techniques. M-mode gives excellent resolution and allows measurement of LV dimensions and wall thickness. 2-D techniques are often used to provide a visual assessment of LV systolic function, both regional and global. The general validity of this has been shown but there are inter-observer variations. Visual estimation is clinically useful but unreliable in those who have poor echo images, can be limited in value in serial evaluation and inadequate where LV volumes critically influence the timing of intervention. Computer software on the echo machine may be used to provide a quantitative assessment of LV function. Certain geometrical assumptions are made about LV shape which are not always valid, particularly in the diseased heart.

M-mode (Fig. 4.1) can be used to assess LV cavity dimensions, wall motion and thickness. The phrase, 'a big heart is a bad heart', carries an important

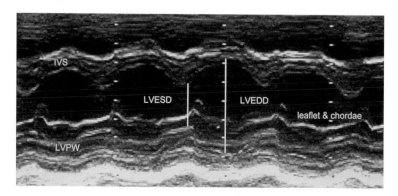

Fig. 4.1 *M-mode of left ventricle. This can be used to estimate cavity dimensions in systole and diastole, and wall thickness. It is important to identify the continuous endocardial echo and to distinguish this from echoes from chordae or mitral valve leaflet tips.*

element of truth – poor LV systolic function is usually associated with increased LV dimensions. This is not always the case, e.g. if there is a large akinetic segment of LV wall or an apical LV aneurysm following MI, systolic function may be impaired due to regional wall motion abnormalities but M-mode measurements of LV dimensions may be within the normal range.

LV internal dimension measurements in end-systole (LVESD) and end-diastole (LVEDD) are made at the level of the MV leaflet tips in the parasternal long-axis view. Measurements are taken from the endocardium of the left surface of the interventricular septum (IVS) to the endocardium of the LV posterior wall (LVPW). The ultrasound beam should be as perpendicular as possible to the IVS. Care must be taken to distinguish between the endocardial surfaces and the chordae tendineae on the M-mode tracing.

LVEDD is at the end of diastole (R wave of ECG). The normal range is 3.5–5.6 cm.

LVESD is at the end of systole, which occurs at the peak downward motion of the IVS (which usually slightly precedes the peak upward motion of the LVPW) and coincides with the T wave on the ECG. The normal range is 2.0–4.0 cm.

Remember that the normal range for LVEDD and LVESD varies with a number of factors, including height, sex and age.

M-mode measurements can be converted to estimates of volume but this is inaccurate in regional LV dysfunction and spherical ventricles. The LVEDD and LVESD measurements can be used to calculate LV fractional shortening, LV ejection fraction and LV volume, which give some further indication of LV systolic function.

Fractional shortening (FS) is a commonly used measure and is the % change in LV internal dimensions (not volumes) between systole and diastole:

$$FS = \frac{LVEDD - LVESD}{LVEDD} \times 100\%$$

Normal range is 30–45%.

The LV volume is derived from the 'cubed equation' (i.e. volume, $V = D^3$, where D is the ventricular dimension measured by M-mode). This assumes that the LV cavity is an ellipse shape, which is not always correct. There are some equations which attempt to improve the accuracy of this technique. The volume in end-diastole is estimated as $(LVEDD)^3$ and in end-systole as $(LVESD)^3$. The **ejection fraction (EF)** is the % change in LV volume between systole and diastole and is:

$$EF = \frac{(LVEDD)^3 - (LVESD)^3}{(LVEDD)^3} \times 100\%$$

Normal range is 50–85%.

LV wall motion and changes in thickness during systole can be measured. The IVS moves towards the LVPW and the amplitude of this motion can be used as an indicator of LV function.

Wall thickness can also be measured. The walls thicken during systole. The normal range of thickness is 6–12 mm. Walls thinner than 6 mm may be stretched as in dilated cardiomyopathy or scarred and damaged by previous MI. Walls of thickness over 12 mm may indicate LV hypertrophy, an important independent prognostic factor in cardiovascular outcome risk.

2-D echo can be used qualitatively to assess LV systolic function by viewing the LV in a number of different planes and views. An experienced echo operator can often give a reasonably good visual assessment of LV systolic function as being normal, mildly, moderately or severely impaired, and whether abnormalities are global or regional.

2-D echo can also be used to estimate LV volumes and EF. Multiple algorithms may be used to estimate LV volumes from 2-D images but all make some geometrical assumptions which may be invalid. The area–length method (symmetrical ventricles) and the apical biplane summation of discs method (asymmetrical ventricles) are validated and normal values available.

A number of techniques are available. Simpson's method (Fig. 4.2) divides the LV cavity into multiple slices of known thickness and diameter D (by taking multiple short-axis views at different levels along the LV long axis) and then calculating the volume of each slice (area × thickness). The area is $\pi(D/2)^2$. The thinner the slices, the more accurate the estimate of LV volume. Calculations can be made by the computer of most echo machines. The endocardial border must be traced accurately and this is often the major technical difficulty. Endocardial definition has improved with some newer echo technology (e.g. harmonic imaging) and automated endocardial border detection systems are available on some echo machines. The computer calculates LV volume by dividing the apical view into 20 sections along the LV long axis.

The LV ejection fraction can be obtained from LV volumes in systole and diastole (as above). Alternatively, computer-derived data can be obtained by taking and tracing the LV endocardial borders of a systolic and a diastolic LV frame.

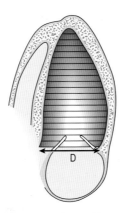

Fig. 4.2 *Simpson's method to estimate left ventricular volume.*

An estimate of cardiac output can be obtained using LV volumes:

Cardiac output = stroke volume × heart rate

Stroke volume = LV diastolic volume − LV systolic volume.

Measurements of LV shape are an important and underutilized aspect of LV remodelling, e.g. after MI. Increasing LV sphericity has prognostic importance and loss of the normal LV shape may be an early indicator of LV dysfunction. 2-D echo allows a simple assessment of LV shape (measuring the ratio of long axis length to mid-cavity diameter).

The location and extent of wall motion abnormality following MI correlates with LV EF and is prognostically useful.

Regional LV wall motion

The LV can be divided up on 2-D imaging of apical 4-chamber and parasternal short-axis views into segments (9 or 16) and an assessment can be made of these segments (Fig. 5.12). This can be useful at rest and in stress echo to determine the location of coronary artery disease (Ch. 5).

A segment's systolic movement may be classified as:

- Normal
- Hypokinetic (reduced movement)

- Akinetic (absent movement)
- Dyskinetic (movement in the wrong direction, e.g. outwards movement of the LV free wall during LV systole)
- Aneurysmal (out-pouching of all layers of the wall).

4.3 CORONARY ARTERY DISEASE

Echo plays an increasingly important role in assessing coronary artery disease. Resting and stress echo (Ch. 5) techniques are used in:

- Assessment of extent of ischaemia or infarction
- Prediction of artery causing ischaemia
- MI – LV function acutely and post MI, ischaemic cardiomyopathy
- RV infarction
- Complications of MI – MR, VSD, mural thrombus, LV aneurysm, pseudoaneurysm, effusion, rupture
- Coronary artery abnormalities, e.g. aneurysm, anomalous origin by transthoracic echo and TOE
- Chest pain with normal coronaries – AS, HCM, MV prolapse.

Assessment of ischaemia

Ischaemia results in immediate changes which can be detected by echo:

- Abnormalities of wall motion (hypokinetic, akinetic, dyskinetic)*
- Abnormalities of wall thickening (reduced or absent systolic thickening or systolic thinning – this is more sensitive and specific for ischaemia)*
- Abnormalities of overall LV function (e.g. ejection fraction).

(* also known as asynergy)

These can be detected by 2-D echo but M-mode is also extremely good because its high sampling rate makes it very sensitive to wall motion and thickening abnormalities. It is essential that the beam is at 90° to the wall. There are limited regions of the LV myocardium that can be examined by M-mode – most usefully, the posterior wall and IVS (Fig. 4.3).

The changes reverse if ischaemia is reversed, e.g. by rest, anti-anginal medication, percutaneous transluminal coronary angioplasty, thrombolysis or coronary artery bypass grafting. If the myocardium has its blood supply occluded for more than 1 h, permanent changes occur which include MI and scarring.

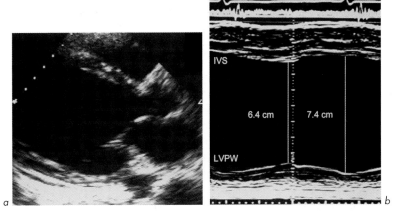

Fig. 4.3 (a) and **(b)** *Dilated left ventricle with impaired systolic function due to coronary artery disease.*

Prediction of artery involved

This is done by dividing the LV into segments as described (Figs 5.12 and 5.13). Stress echo is based on this.

Assessment of myocardial infarction

Echo can help in detecting the extent of LV infarction, assessing RV involvement and detecting complications. The changes in LV function with acute MI are similar to those described for ischaemia, but rapidly become irreversible. Detection of RV involvement is important in determining treatment and prognosis (section 4.6).

Complications of myocardial infarction

Many of the complications of acute MI can be detected by echo.

- **Acute heart failure due to extensive MI.** This leads to pump failure which may result in cardiogenic shock. Echo shows severe LV impairment.

75

In the following 2 complications (acute MR and acute VSD), LV systolic function is very active, unlike the situation above.

- **Acute MR.** This may be due to papillary muscle dysfunction or rupture (Fig. 4.4) or chordal rupture, which may be shown by 2-D echo. There may be a flail MV leaflet. The MR jet can be seen on continuous wave or colour flow mapping.

- **Acute VSD.** This is often near the cardiac apex and is more common in inferior and RV infarction. A discontinuity in the IVS can be seen on 2-D echo in the apical 4-chamber, parasternal long-axis and short-axis views. Colour flow mapping can show the defect. Pulsed wave Doppler moved along the RV side of the IVS (parasternal long-axis or sometimes 4-chamber views) can show the jet.

- **Mural thrombus** (Fig. 4.5). This is shown on 2-D echo. It is usually located near an infarcted segment or aneurysm.

- **LV aneurysm.** Most frequently seen at or near the apex. More common in anterior than inferior MI. Best seen on 2-D echo. These can vary in size from small to very large, sometimes larger than the LV.

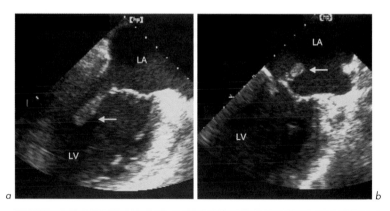

a   b

Fig. 4.4 (a) and **(b)** *Papillary muscle rupture following acute myocardial infarction. The muscle (arrows) and the posterior mitral valve leaflet can be seen to prolapse into the left atrium. TOE study.*

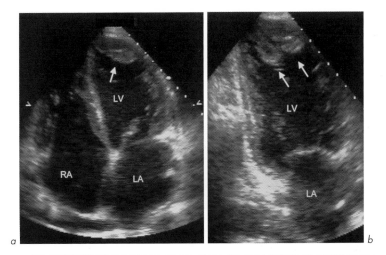

Fig. 4.5 *Thrombus in the apex of the left ventricle (arrows) following myocardial infarction. (**a**) Apical 4-chamber view and (**b**) apical 2-chamber view showing 2 distinct masses.*

- **Pseudoaneurysm (false aneurysm).** This is rare. It follows rupture of the LV free wall and leads to haemopericardium (blood in the pericardial space), tamponade and is usually rapidly fatal. Sometimes, the haemopericardium clots and seals off the hole in the LV and a false aneurysm forms. 2-D echo is a good way to diagnose this. It is important to detect, as it needs urgent surgical resection before it ruptures. It can be difficult to distinguish it from a true aneurysm but the communicating neck is usually narrower than the diameter of the aneurysm, the walls are thinner and its size changes in the cardiac cycle (expands in systole) and it is more often filled with thrombus.

- **Pericardial effusion** complicating MI can be detected by M-mode or 2-D echo.

- **Myocardial function after MI.** This gives an indication of prognosis. The scarred myocardium is seen as a thin segment which does not thicken during systole and has abnormal motion. Echo can assess the extent of MI, evaluate LV systolic and diastolic function and look at residual complications.

Myocardial 'hibernation' and 'stunning'

The heart is critically dependent upon its blood supply. Occlusion of a coronary artery results in the cessation of myocardial contraction within 1 min. Myocardial cell death usually occurs after 15 min of ischaemia.

An impairment of contractile function may remain even after restoration of the blood supply without MI. This effect has been termed *myocardial stunning* (stunned heart). It may cause reversible systolic or diastolic dysfunction. Although stunned myocardium is viable, normal function may not be regained for up to 2 weeks. Recurrent episodes of ischaemia may result in the loss of normal function of the heart, and the term *hibernating myocardium* (hibernation) has been applied to a similar condition.

Echo assessment of coronary artery anatomy (Fig. 4.6)

Echo is not yet able to give a very accurate assessment of most parts of the coronary anatomy. The origins of the left and right coronary arteries may be seen in some transthoracic echo studies by using a modified parasternal short-axis view at AV level.

Abnormalities are more likely to be seen during TOE, e.g.

- Anomalous origin of coronaries (e.g. origin from PA)
- Coronary artery fistula
- Aneurysm, e.g. Kawasaki syndrome, an acquired condition in children with coronary aneurysms which may be several centimetres in diameter.

Useful information from echo in patients with heart failure

Left ventricle

- Dimensions – systolic and diastolic
- Systolic function and an indication of fractional shortening and ejection fraction
- Regional or global wall motion abnormalities – evidence of previous infarction, ischaemia or aneurysm
- Wall thickness – concentric hypertrophy (e.g. hypertension or amyloid) or asymmetrical hypertrophy (e.g. HCM)
- Evidence of diastolic heart failure.

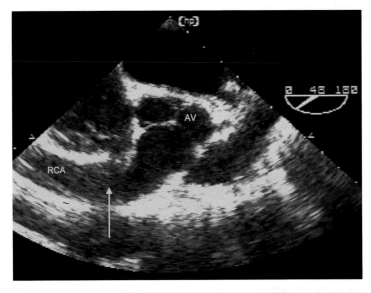

Fig. 4.6 *Huge dilatation of the right coronary artery (RCA, arrow) due to coronary fistula. TOE short-axis study at aortic valve level.*

Valves

- Aortic stenosis or regurgitation
- Mitral regurgitation – as a cause of heart failure or secondary to ventricular dilatation ('functional')
- Mitral stenosis.

Pericardium

- Effusion
- Constriction
- Echo suggestion of cardiac tamponade (e.g. RV diastolic collapse).

Right heart

- Right ventricular dimensions
- PHT (estimation of PASP by Doppler assessment of TR).

Left atrium
- Dimensions (particularly if AF and planned cardioversion).

Intracardiac thrombus

Changes in heart size and function in response to therapy

4.4 CARDIOMYOPATHIES AND MYOCARDITIS

The cardiomyopathies are a diverse group of disorders. Cardiomyopathy means heart muscle abnormality, and strictly speaking the term should be applied to conditions that have no known underlying cause. These are known as idiopathic cardiomyopathies. The term has been extended to include conditions where there is an underlying cause (e.g. alcoholic, ischaemic, hypertensive cardiomyopathy etc.)

The most important idiopathic cardiomyopathies are:
- Hypertrophic (increased ventricular wall thickness)
- Dilated (increased ventricular volume)
- Restrictive (increased ventricular stiffness).

1. Hypertrophic cardiomyopathy

This is an autosomal dominant condition with a high mutation rate (up to 50% of cases are sporadic). It is rare with an incidence of 0.4 –2.5 per 100 000 per year. A number of mutations of cardiac proteins have been identified as underlying causes. These include β-myosin heavy chain, myosin-binding protein C, α-tropomyosin and troponin T.

The clinical features include:
- Angina with normal coronary arteries – due to ventricular hypertrophy and myocardial oxygen supply/demand imbalance)
- Arrhythmias
- Breathlessness
- Syncope
- Sudden cardiac death (annual death rate is 3% in adults) – due to outflow tract obstruction or arrhythmia
- Ejection systolic murmur which may be confused with valvular aortic stenosis
- Heart failure (10–15%).

The characteristic feature is myocardial hypertrophy in any part of the ventricular wall:

- IVS to a greater extent than the free wall (termed asymmetrical septal hypertrophy or ASH) – 60% of cases
- Concentric – 30% of cases
- Apical – 10% of cases
- RV hypertrophy – 30% of cases and correlates with severity of LVH.

Hypertrophy, particularly of the septum, may cause LV outflow tract obstruction (LVOTO). In this situation, the term hypertrophic *obstructive* cardiomyopathy (HOCM) is appropriate. This 'dynamic' obstruction becomes more pronounced in the later stages of systole. As the LV empties, LV cavity size becomes smaller and the anterior MV leaflet moves anteriorly to contact the septum. It may be present at rest or become more pronounced with exercise. In some individuals with HCM, the most dangerous time is at the end of vigorous exercise, e.g. at half-time in a football match. At this time, ventricular volumes diminish as cardiac output and heart rate decrease, catecholamine drive decreases and there may be changes in circulating electrolyte concentrations, such as K^+. These features all combine to increase the risk of syncope and sudden death by increasing the likelihood of LVOTO and arrhythmias.

Echo is diagnostic of HCM. The important echo features are seen using both **M-mode** and **2-D imaging**:

1. Asymmetrical septal hypertrophy (ASH) (Fig. 4.7)
2. Systolic anterior motion (SAM) of the MV apparatus which may abut the IVS. This may not be seen at rest but may occur following provocation by the Valsalva manoeuvre or isovolumic exercise
3. Midsystolic AV closure and fluttering.

The definition of asymmetrical hypertrophy varies but a septal to posterior wall ratio of 1.5 or more is unequivocal evidence of asymmetry.

Neither ASH nor SAM is specific for HCM. ASH may occur in AS and SAM may occur in MV prolapse. Their occurrence together is strongly suggestive of HCM.

Continuous wave Doppler shows increased peak flow through the LVOT. Pulsed wave Doppler with the sample volume in the LVOT proximal to the AV shows that the increase in velocity occurs below the level of the valve, distinguishing the obstruction from valvular aortic stenosis. The peak in maximal

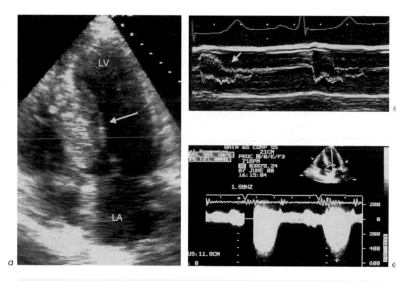

a

Fig. 4.7 *Hypertrophic cardiomyopathy.* **(a)** *Asymmetrical septal hypertrophy (arrow).* **(b)** *Fluttering and premature mid-systolic closure of the aortic valve (arrow).* **(c)** *Continuous Doppler showing a peak velocity across the left ventricular outflow tract of 5.6 m/s (estimated peak gradient 127 mmHg).*

velocity across the AV is often bifid in HCM. There may also be features of LV diastolic dysfunction due to LVH (e.g. abnormal transmitral flow pattern with E-wave smaller than A-wave, section 4.5).

2. Dilated cardiomyopathy

This is characterized by dilatation of the cardiac chambers, particularly the LV (although all other chambers are often involved) with reduced wall thickness and reduced wall motion (Fig. 4.8). The incidence is estimated at 6.0 per 100 000 per year. Most cases are isolated although some familial forms have been identified. The reduced LV wall motion is usually global rather than regional, as seen in LV systolic impairment due to coronary artery disease (ischaemia or infarction).

M-mode and **2-D echo** show:
- Dilatation of all the cardiac chambers (left and right ventricles and atria) – increased LVESD and LVEDD

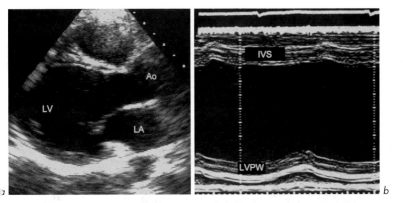

Fig. 4.8 (a) and **(b)** *Dilated left ventricle with impaired systolic function due to dilated cardiomyopathy. Parasternal long-axis view and M-mode.*

- Reduced wall thickness and motion (ranging from mild to severe impairment) – reduced ejection fraction and fractional shortening, reduced motion of IVS and LVPW
- Intracardiac thrombus (LV and LA).

Doppler studies may show functional MR and TR.

A number of conditions give rise to a clinical picture which is similar to idiopathic dilated cardiomyopathy. These include toxins such as alcohol and certain drugs, especially those used in the treatment of some cancers.

Chemotherapy with **doxorubicin** produces a dose-dependent degenerative cardiomyopathy. Cumulative doses should be kept to below 450–500 mg/m². Subtle abnormalities of LV systolic function (increased wall stress) are found in approximately 1 in 6 patients receiving only one dose of doxorubicin. Most patients who receive at least 228 mg/m² show either reduced contractility or increased wall stress. Baseline and re-evaluation echo should be carried out in individuals receiving doxorubicin. Further administration appears to be safe if resting EF remains normal, and dangerous if EF is low. Early abnormalities of diastolic function (in the absence of systolic abnormalities) may occur in patients receiving 200–300 mg/m².

3. Restrictive cardiomyopathy

This is characterized by increased myocardial stiffness or impaired relaxation and abnormal diastolic function of one or both ventricles. A number of disorders give rise to a clinical picture of restrictive cardiomyopathy:

1. Idiopathic
2. Infiltrations – amyloid, sarcoid, haemochromatosis, glycogen storage diseases (e.g. Pompe's), mucopolysaccharidoses (e.g. Gaucher's, Fabry's)
3. Endomyocardial fibrosis – hypereosinophilic syndrome (Loeffler's endomyocardial fibrosis), carcinoid, malignancy.

The echo assessment is difficult and the features are not specific. If features of restrictive cardiomyopathy are present, evidence of myocardial infiltration or endomyocardial fibrosis should be sought. The echo differentiation between restrictive cardiomyopathy and constrictive pericarditis can be difficult but is important as it has management implications.

Echo features of restrictive cardiomyopathy

- LV and RV cavity sizes are usually normal or only mildly increased, but there is impaired contractility of the ventricular walls seen on M-mode and 2-D echo. There may be dilatation of the LA and RA.
- Impaired LV and RV diastolic function. This is best assessed by Doppler echo. There is often a characteristic abnormal 'restrictive pattern' of MV flow with a very large E-wave and small A-wave (section 4.5).

Infiltration

The findings are similar whatever the underlying cause. Amyloid is the most common infiltrative disease (Fig. 4.9). The features are:

- Concentric thickening of the LV and RV free walls and septum and the interatrial septum
- LV and RV internal dimensions are often reduced
- Reduced wall and septal motion
- Failure of systolic thickening of the IVS and LV free wall
- Patches of high intensity 'speckling' in the hypertrophied muscle
- Thickening of the MV and TV leaflets with regurgitation (aortic and pulmonary valves may also be thickened)
- Pericardial effusion

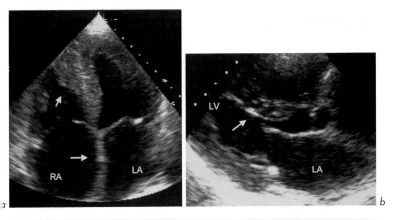

Fig. 4.9 Amyloid heart disease. **(a)** There is left ventricular and right ventricular hypertrophy, with apical obliteration of the right ventricle cavity with thrombus (arrow). The atria are dilated and the interatrial septum is thickened (arrow), as are the valve leaflets. **(b)** Hypertrophy and speckling of the interventricular septum (arrow).

- LV diastolic impairment with or without systolic impairment
- Intracardiac thrombus.

Endomyocardial fibrosis

- Cavity obliteration especially at the RV and LV apex due to fibrosis or eosinophilic infiltration
- Bright echogenic endocardium
- Normal or thickened LV walls with reduced contractility
- Normal LV or reduced cavity size
- Similar changes in RV to LV
- Dilated RA and LA
- Intracardiac thrombus
- LV diastolic impairment with or without systolic impairment.

4. Myocarditis

This is inflammation of the heart muscle. The underlying cause is often not found, or it may be due to:

- Viruses such as Coxsackie B, influenza
- Bacteria such as *Mycoplasma pneumoniae*
- Parasites, e.g. Chagas' disease, Lyme disease (section 7.8)
- Toxins, e.g. ethanol, drugs, chemicals
- Connective tissue disease, e.g. SLE
- Fungi.

This is a clinical diagnosis and there may be a history suggestive of an underlying cause. The ECG often shows a resting tachycardia with widespread T-wave inversion. The echo features are not specific and are similar to those of dilated cardiomyopathy, with impaired systolic and diastolic function and evidence of new valvular regurgitation (e.g. MR). Serial echo examinations may show a change in LV function or valvular abnormalities which would support the diagnosis of myocarditis rather than dilated cardiomyopathy. There may be regional LV wall motion abnormalities in myocarditis.

4.5 DIASTOLIC FUNCTION

Clinical features of left heart failure may occur in individuals with normal or near-normal LV systolic function assessed by echo, due to diastolic dysfunction, systolic impairment on exertion or ischaemia.

Diastolic function of the LV relates to chamber stiffness and relaxation following ventricular contraction. It is not a passive phenomenon and requires energy. Abnormalities of LV diastolic function occur in a number of conditions and can be assessed by echo but their assessment is rather complex. These abnormalities may co-exist with abnormalities of systolic function, or may occur in isolation or before systolic impairment becomes obvious.

Diastole has 4 periods – isovolumic relaxation, early rapid filling, late filling and atrial systole. Abnormalities in any of these may contribute to diastolic heart failure.

Heart failure may be predominantly diastolic in one-third of cases. In these cases, echo measures of diastolic function can be abnormal. It is wise to assess LV systolic and diastolic function separately since the causes of abnormalities and, more importantly, their treatments, differ.

Diastolic heart failure is common in the elderly and should be suspected in patients with symptoms of heart failure with normal size hearts and ventricular hypertrophy and/or myocardial ischaemia. Diastolic heart failure occurs in up to 50% of patients with heart failure in the community but is less common (<10%) in those admitted to hospital with heart failure.

Causes of LV diastolic impairment

These often co-exist (e.g. hypertension and coronary artery disease):
1. Ageing effects
2. LV hypertrophy – hypertension, AS, HCM
3. Ischaemic heart disease
4. Restrictive cardiomyopathy
5. LV infiltrations – amyloid, sarcoid, carcinoid, haemochromatosis
6. Pericardial constriction.

In general, these are conditions which increase stiffness of the LV wall. LV relaxation is then abnormal, impairing diastolic flow from LA into LV. Diastolic function is more sensitive than systolic function to the effects of age and is very dependent on filling conditions.

Remember that from Newton's second law of motion (force = mass × acceleration), the only factor that causes blood to move from LA to LV is atrioventricular force (or pressure gradient, in mmHg/cm). Ventricular disease modifies diastolic LV filling by modifying this gradient. Blood acceleration, not blood velocity, is proportional to the atrioventricular pressure gradient. Peak blood velocity thus depends not only on the peak pressure gradient but also on the time during which it has acted.

Echo assessment of LV diastolic function

LV diastolic function is complex and dependent upon a number of factors such as age, preload, afterload, heart rate and the co-existence of other abnormalities (e.g. MV disease).

There is no good single echo measure. Doppler measurements of LV filling pattern should not necessarily be viewed as the only reflection of LV 'diastolic function'. It is a mistake to rely on single measurements such as E:A ratios (see below) and many anatomical and haemodynamic features should be considered together.

Surgically correctable conditions which mimic diastolic dysfunction such as constrictive pericarditis must be excluded by echo and, if necessary, other techniques such as magnetic resonance imaging (MRI), computed tomography (CT) scanning and cardiac catheterization.

Using **M-mode**, motion of the anterior mitral valve leaflet (AMVL) during diastole has a characteristic M-shaped (E–A) pattern, assuming that the individual is in sinus rhythm and there is no MS. If the LV is stiffer than usual, abnormalities of AMVL motion may be observed, e.g.:

- Diminished AMVL excursion (E-wave)
- Increase in A-wave size (as atrial contraction contributes to a greater extent to diastolic filling of the LV)
- Reduced E:A ratio.

These are *not* specific or highly sensitive for LV diastolic impairment.

The normal LV myocardium relaxes without any increase in LV volume during the interval between closure of the AV (A_2) and opening of the MV. This is called the isovolumic relaxation time (IVRT) and is usually 50–80 ms. The IVRT often increases with diastolic dysfunction, but also normally increases with age (see below).

2-D echo does not help to make a direct assessment of LV diastolic dysfunction but can detect associated abnormalities such as:

- LV hypertrophy
- Myocardial infiltration (e.g. amyloid)
- Pericardial effusion and/or thickening
- Ischaemic heart disease (regional LV wall motion and thickening abnormalities or scarring)
- Dilated IVC
- **There may also be co-existent LV systolic abnormalities.**

Doppler can provide useful information regarding LV diastolic dysfunction but relying on measures of transmitral flow alone is not sufficient.

IVRT often increases with diastolic dysfunction, but also increases with age and changes with heart rate. Impaired relaxation is thus associated with a prolonged IVRT, whilst decreased compliance and elevated filling pressures are associated with a shortened IVRT. Thus, IVRT measurement is useful in determining the severity of diastolic dysfunction, particularly in serial studies of patients to assess response to medical therapy or disease progression. IVRT is measured from an apical 4-chamber view angulated anteriorly to show the

LVOT and AV. Using pulsed wave Doppler, a 3–5 mm sample volume is positioned midway between the AV and MV to obtain a signal showing both aortic outflow and mitral inflow, ideally with a defined AV closing click. IVRT is measured as the time from the middle of the aortic closure click to the onset of mitral flow.

The MV diastolic flow pattern reflects flow into the LV. This can be assessed by pulsed Doppler using the apical 4-chamber view with the sample volume in the mitral orifice.

Mitral flow pattern is influenced by a large number of factors. These include LV stiffness, preload, afterload, cardiac rhythm, conduction abnormalities, LA systolic function, heart rate, AR, MR and the phase of respiration.

In the normal heart, there is a characteristic flow pattern:

- The E-wave is the result of passive early diastolic LV filling.
- The A-wave represents active late diastolic LV filling due to LA contraction.
- The acceleration time (AT) and deceleration time (DT) of the E-wave can be measured. AT is the time from onset of diastolic flow to the peak of the E-wave. DT is the time from the E-wave peak to the point where the deceleration slope hits the baseline.

The E-wave is often greater than the A-wave but it is important to remember that this **varies with age**. The E-wave, E:A ratio and E-wave deceleration times tend to fall with increasing age.

Age- and gender-specific normal ranges for mitral flow-derived indices of LV diastolic function in a general population have been published. Approximate values are:

	Men	Women
Peak E-wave (m/s)	0.66 ± 0.15	0.70 ± 0.16
E-wave deceleration time (s)	0.21 ± 0.04	0.19 ± 0.04
Peak A-wave (m/s)	0.67 ± 0.16	0.72 ± 0.18
E:A ratio	1.04 ± 0.38	1.03 ± 0.34

(Data from Tromsø Study, Eur Heart J 2000; 21:1376–1386.)

Two abnormal mitral flow patterns are recognized (Figs 4.10, 4.11):

1. **'Slow-relaxation pattern'.** Decreased LV relaxation due to diastolic dysfunction associated with LV hypertrophy or myocardial ischaemia:
   - E-wave is small, A-wave is large, AT prolonged, IVRT prolonged.
2. **'Restrictive pattern'.** Reduced LV filling may be caused by restrictive cardiomyopathy or constrictive pericarditis (conditions causing a rapid rise of LV diastolic pressure). It may, however, occur in other conditions such as with high LV filling pressures, systolic heart failure, MR, HCM:
   - E-wave very tall, A-wave is small, DT short, IVRT short.

Other echo methods to assess diastolic function

These include 'acoustic quantification' available on some echo machines. Using automatic border detection software, the endocardial border of the LV can be continuously outlined on a 4-chamber view. This can produce LV area/time and LV volume/time curves. Abnormalities of these diastolic filling parameters can be detected even when the mitral Doppler flow pattern is normal and this appears to be a sensitive technique to detect early diastolic dysfunction.

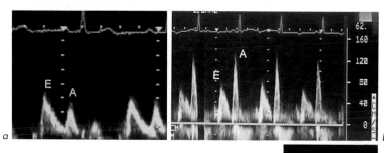

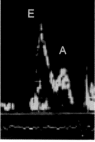

Fig. 4.10 *Mitral flow patterns on pulsed wave Doppler.*
(a) Normal; (b) tall A-wave; (c) tall E-wave.

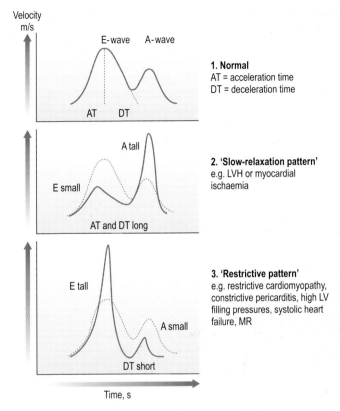

Fig. 4.11 *Mitral valve flow patterns.*

Myocardial tissue Doppler imaging (TDI)

During diastolic LV filling, the myocardial walls move outwards. The amplitude, pattern and velocity of this motion can be recorded using pulsed wave tissue Doppler imaging (TDI). This is an important method of identifying and quantifying myocardial mechanics. The velocity scale, wall filters and gain of the echo machine are adjusted to display the Doppler velocities of the movement of the myocardium, which are lower than intracavity blood flow velocities. These velocities are less dependent upon preload and are useful, in addition to Doppler

91

transmitral flow, in evaluating diastolic function. Signals are recorded using pulsed wave Doppler in an apical 4-chamber view in a small sample volume of 2–3 mm positioned in the myocardium of the basal LV wall, about 1 cm from the mitral annulus. Signals may be recorded from the basal septum or basal lateral wall although the septal signals tend to be more reproducible. The velocity scale is decreased to a range of only around 0.2 m/s and the wall filters are reduced to obtain a well-defined signal. Some echo machines have a tissue Doppler setting that automatically makes these adjustments. Recordings are made at end expiration during normal quiet respiration.

The cardiac cycle can be divided into time intervals based upon mechanical events: filling and ejection. There are also isovolumic intervals before and after ejection. During ejection, there is a positive systolic myocardial wave towards the transducer (S_m). The filling period has 2 elements – E_m and A_m (Fig. 4.12). The pattern of myocardial motion is similar but inverted and lower in velocity compared to transmitral flows. When myocardial tissue Doppler velocities are recorded from the mitral annulus using an apical approach, there is a brief early velocity away from the transducer corresponding to early diastolic relaxation with a velocity of 8–12 cm/s. This is called the early myocardial velocity (E_m). Following atrial contraction, a second velocity wave away from the apex is seen, the atrial myocardial velocity (A_m), usually 4–8 cm/s. The normal ratio of E_m to A_m is over 1.0. A reduced E_m to A_m ratio indicates impaired relaxation. The pattern of E_m to A_m also helps to distinguish normal LV filling from the pseudonormalization pattern seen in patients suffering from moderate to severe diastolic dysfunction.

Approximate values for TDI-derived variables and IVRT are:

- E_m 10.3 ± 2.0 cm/s
- A_m 5.8 ± 1.6 cm/s
- E_m/A_m 2.1 ± 0.9
- IVRT 63 ± 11 ms

Athletic heart and screening before exercise

Vigorous athletic training is associated with several physiological and biochemical adaptations which enable an increase in cardiac output. An increase in cardiac chamber size is fundamental to the generation of a sustained increase in cardiac output for prolonged periods. Echo studies have shown that the vast majority of

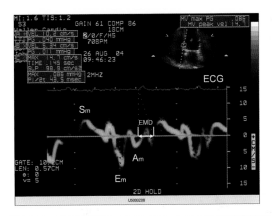

Fig. 4.12 Myocardial tissue Doppler imaging (TDI). Apical 4-chamber view showing septal motion. Sm = systolic, Em = early, Am = atrial myocardial velocities. EMD = electro-mechanical delay.

athletes have modest cardiac enlargement although a small proportion exhibit substantial increases. Training results in compensated changes in cardiac anatomy, primarily of the LV, leading to the development of an 'athletic heart'. This does not occur in casual recreational athletes, as substantial training is needed for this to develop. The major determinants of cardiac morphological adaptation to training include body size (body surface area or height) and participation in certain endurance sports such as skiing, cycling, running and canoeing. Cardiac dimensions vary considerably amongst athletes, even when allowances are made for these variables, suggesting that genetic, endocrine and biochemical factors also influence heart size.

The type of athletic activity impacts on the nature of LV remodelling. In general, 2 main types of adaptation are recognized:

- LV chamber enlargement. Vigorous endurance training, e.g. long distance running/cycling/skiing/canoeing leads to an endurance type of elevation in LV mass due to LV chamber enlargement and, to a lesser degree, an increase in wall thickness and mild LVH.
- Left ventricular hypertrophy. Intense isotonic training (e.g. weight lifting) leads to a 'strength type' concentric LVH.

Note that many athletes use a combination of these endurance and strengthening training techniques, so these 'pure' categories of athletic heart are rare and most have a combination. Some individuals involved in intense competition have used anabolic steroid supplements, which can cause significant pathological LVH.

The clinical **echo** differentiation of athletic heart from other causes of LVH such as HCM can be difficult but may be helped by the following points:

- In general, in males with an athletic heart, LV posterior wall diastolic thickness is rarely over 13 mm (it may be 13–16 mm in approximately 2% of male athletes).
- The posterior wall thickness to LV diameter ratio remains normal.
- LV posterior wall thickness of over 16 mm has not been reported due to athletic heart alone and should raise the possibility of HCM.
- The differentiation between athletic heart and pathological LVH is less difficult in female athletes, as LV wall thickness in elite female athletes is 6–12 mm (in the normal range) and so increased wall thickness is likely to be abnormal.
- Other ways to differentiate athletic heart from pathological hypertrophy include examining diastolic function using transmitral E to A ratios, tissue Doppler imaging for peak E_m wave velocity, which is high over the septum and lateral wall in athletes (over 8 cm/s), and tissue strain imaging.

Tests other than echo may be carried out. Measurement of maximum oxygen consumption during exercise (MVO_2) is useful and is supranormal in those with athletic hearts relative to those with HCM.

Screening and echo before exercise

Before undertaking competitive athletic activities in many countries, individuals are advised to undergo a general health evaluation. From the cardiovascular viewpoint, this means a full clinical history (e.g. of any cardiac symptoms including a family history of HCM or sudden death) and a full examination including blood pressure, pulse and cardiovascular examination. Further investigation may include ECG, exercise ECG and echo. With no symptoms or family history and a normal examination, the chance of finding significant heart disease, likely to affect exercise capacity, is very low. Echo may, in these patients, have a low yield. **Echo** should be performed if there is:

- History of exertional syncope
- Family history of sudden cardiac death or HCM
- Murmur suggestive of HCM or AS.

Screening of athletes

In some countries, an echo is recommended for all professional athletes.

Screening for relevant conditions which may cause LVOTO, e.g. HOCM or AS, should be detected by clinical assessments. Disease of the proximal aorta or occult valve diseases are rare. Echo can, in some cases, identify the origin of both coronary arteries. This is important as anomalous origins of coronary arteries have been associated with sudden death during exercise.

Conditions increasing the risk of exercise which may be detected by echo

High/moderate risk:

- HOCM
- Aortic dilatation, e.g. Marfan's
- Valvular AS (severe or moderate)
- Occult dilated cardiomyopathy
- PHT
- Anomalous origin of the coronary arteries.

Low risk:

- MV prolapse with mild MR
- Mild AS such as bicuspid AV with a Doppler gradient of under 36 mmHg
- Mild MS
- Mild PS
- Uncomplicated ASD
- Small restrictive VSD.

4.6 RIGHT HEART AND LUNGS

Right ventricular (RV) function

RV function plays a critical role in a number of congenital and acquired cardiac conditions. Accurate measurement of RV function is important in planning treatment and predicting prognosis. Until recently, RV function has attracted less attention than LV function. The main reasons have been a lack of understanding of its important role in the circulation and difficulties in assessing its function due to its complex anatomy.

Echo plays a role in assessing RV volume and function but is often used in combination with other modalities such as contrast ventriculography, radionuclide ventriculography, ultrafast CT and MRI. Even more accurate assessment can be made by the construction of RV pressure-volume loops (usually using data from cardiac catheterization).

Clinical importance of RV function

1. Myocardial infarction

RV dysfunction is well recognized in MI. Anterior MI is usually associated with persistent LV regional impairment and transient global RV impairment, whereas inferior MI is associated with persistent regional impairment in both ventricles. The haemodynamic responses to infarction differ in the RV and LV. In patients with extensive RV infarction, cardiogenic shock is common and requires a different therapeutic approach from LV infarction (Fig. 4.13).

The degree of RV dysfunction can be used to assess prognosis in acute MI. RV ejection fraction is a useful indicator of outcome, and 2-year mortality is higher in patients with a low RV ejection fraction (<35%).

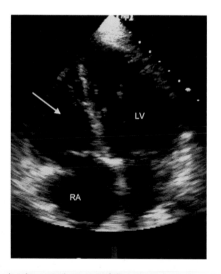

Fig. 4.13 *Dilated right ventricle (arrow) following acute right ventricular infarction. Apical 4-chamber view.*

RV function is also important in predicting the prognosis in patients with VSD following MI. RV dysfunction is a major cause of cardiogenic shock and death in such patients.

2. Valvular heart disease (e.g. MS, PS)

RV function can play an important role in timing surgery.

3. Chronic lung disease causing PHT

RV function plays an important role in the long-term outcome of patients with chronic airflow limitation or pulmonary fibrosis. When such diseases are associated with PHT, RV dilatation and failure (leading to cor pulmonale), they have a poor outlook.

4. Septicaemic shock and post-cardiotomy shock

These are also associated with RV dysfunction, probably as a result of alterations in RV afterload and contractility.

5. Congenital heart disease before and after surgery (e.g. VSD, ASD, complex disease)

Assessment of RV function is of great importance. It is an important prognostic marker in patients with shunts (e.g. VSD, ASD) or complex conditions such as tetralogy of Fallot or transposition of the great arteries.

6. Pericardial effusion

RV diastolic collapse is an important echo indicator of cardiac tamponade.

Echo assessment of RV function

This is difficult because:
1. The RV has greater geometrical complexity than the LV.
2. The RV free wall is heavily trabeculated, making edge recognition difficult.
3. Overlap between RV and other cardiac chambers in some imaging modalities makes reliable volume measurement difficult.
4. The location of the RV directly under the sternum poses specific problems for echo (the ultrasound beam will not penetrate bone).
5. The assessment of the RV is especially difficult in subjects who have had previous thoracic surgery or have chronic lung disease. RV function studies are often vital for them.

Despite such limitations, M-mode and 2-D echo are used to estimate RV size and function. The best echo views for the RV are usually:

- Subcostal 4-chamber
- Apical 4-chamber
- Parasternal short-axis at MV and papillary muscle levels.

Estimates can be made of RV internal dimensions, wall thickness and ejection fraction. RV function is sensitive to myocardial contractility, preload and afterload but also to LV contractility, the contribution of the septum, and to intrapericardial pressure. An analysis of RV function should take all these factors into account and EF *per se* may not be sensitive enough to these factors.

Right-sided failure is associated with a dilated, hypokinetic RV. If the RV is the same size or larger than the LV in all views, it is abnormal.

Note that even in the most experienced hands, adequate echo examination of the RV may be obtained in only approximately 50% of subjects.

Pulmonary hypertension (Fig. 4.14)

This is defined as an abnormal increase in PA pressure above:

- 30/20 mmHg (normal 25/10 mmHg)
- Mean 20 mmHg at rest
- Mean 30 mmHg during exercise.

In those aged over 50 years, PHT is the third most frequent cardiovascular problem after coronary artery disease and systemic hypertension.

Echo is useful in assessing the underlying cause and severity of PHT (Fig. 4.15), but echo examination can be technically more difficult since many of these individuals have underlying lung disease. This is especially true if the lungs are hyperinflated or there is pulmonary fibrosis.

The echo features of PHT

M-mode

- Abnormal M-mode of the pulmonary valve leaflets with absent A-wave or mid-systolic notch
- Dilated RV with normal LV
- Abnormal IVS motion ('right ventricularization' of IVS)
- Underlying cause, e.g. MS (PA systolic pressure is an index of severity).

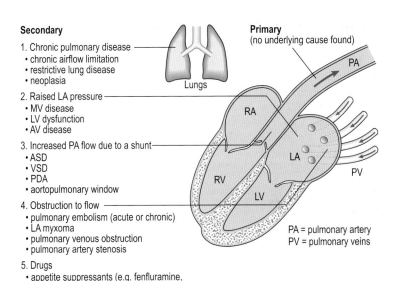

Secondary

1. Chronic pulmonary disease
   • chronic airflow limitation
   • restrictive lung disease
   • neoplasia

2. Raised LA pressure
   • MV disease
   • LV dysfunction
   • AV disease

3. Increased PA flow due to a shunt
   • ASD
   • VSD
   • PDA
   • aortopulmonary window

4. Obstruction to flow
   • pulmonary embolism (acute or chronic)
   • LA myxoma
   • pulmonary venous obstruction
   • pulmonary artery stenosis

5. Drugs
   • appetite suppressants (e.g. fenfluramine, phentermine)

Primary
(no underlying cause found)

PA = pulmonary artery
PV = pulmonary veins

Fig. 4.14 *Schematic representation of causes of pulmonary hypertension.*

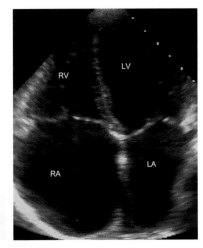

Fig. 4.15 *Pulmonary hypertension. Dilated right atrium and right ventricle in apical 4-chamber view.*

2-D echo

- Dilated PA (e.g. parasternal short-axis view at aortic level). The PA diameter should normally not be greater than aortic diameter
- RV dilatation and/or hypertrophy
- RA dilatation
- Abnormal IVS motion
- Underlying cause, e.g. MV or AV disease, ASD, VSD, LV dysfunction.

Doppler

This is the best method to assess PA systolic pressure using TR velocity (as described in Ch. 3), or short PA acceleration time as a surrogate of PHT.

Pulmonary embolism

Pulmonary embolism (PE) refers to the situation when a mass, usually a blood clot (thrombus) travels in the bloodstream and lodges in the pulmonary arterial system. The origin of the thrombus is usually a systemic vein, often in the legs, pelvis or abdomen. Materials other than thrombus may embolize and include tumours, fat or air. PE is a very common condition and microemboli are found in up to 60% of autopsies, but are diagnosed less frequently in life. Up to 10% of clinically detected PEs are fatal. After PE, lung tissue is ventilated with air but not perfused with blood. This leads to impaired gas exchange and hypoxia (a reduction in the amount of oxygen in the blood). After a few hours, the area of lung involved may collapse and subsequently infarct. The haemodynamic effect of PE is a rise in pulmonary artery pressure and a fall in cardiac output. Echo may help in the diagnosis.

There may be no obvious underlying cause, but the thrombus which may lead to PE can form as a result of:

- Sluggish blood flow
- Local injury
- Venous compression
- Hypercoagulable state.

Risk factors for PE

- Immobility
- Prolonged bed-rest
- Lower limb and pelvic fractures

- Malignancy
- Debilitating systemic diseases, e.g. heart failure
- Pregnancy and childbirth
- Post-surgery, especially abdominal or pelvic
- Inherited hypercoagulable states, e.g. factor V Leiden and deficiency of protein S, protein C or antithrombin III
- Smoking
- Excess oestrogen, e.g. oral contraceptive pill.

Clinical features of PE

There are varied presentations, depending on the size of the PE and the extent of obstruction of the pulmonary circulation. PEs usually present with pleuritic chest pain, dyspnoea, haemoptysis or haemodynamic collapse if there is acute massive PE. The effects of the PE relate to its size and the degree of obstruction in the pulmonary circulation.

There are 4 distinct presentations with different clinical and echo features:

1. **Silent PE**. Many small PEs are not detected clinically.
2. **Small/medium PE**. PE in a terminal pulmonary vessel.
   - Pleuritic chest pain and breathlessness. Haemoptysis in 30% often 3 days or more after PE. May present in a subtle non-specific way with unexplained breathlessness or cough or new-onset AF.
   - Tachypnoea, pleural rub, coarse crackles over area. Fever. Cardiovascular examination may be normal.
   - There may be a blood-stained pleural effusion.
   - Chest X-ray often normal.
   - ECG shows sinus tachycardia, AF, right heart strain if medium-sized PE.
   - Blood tests show raised fibrin degradation products or D-dimer.
   - Other tests may be useful in diagnosis including ultrasound of pelvis and legs, V/Q scan, spiral CT, MRI.
   - **Echo** is usually normal with small PEs. With medium PEs, there may be some echo features of right heart dilatation.
3. **Massive PE**. Rarer. Presents with sudden collapse due to obstruction of RVOT because PE has lodged in main PA.
   - Severe central chest pain (due to myocardial ischaemia caused by reduced coronary arterial flow).
   - May result in shock, syncope due to a sudden reduction in cardiac output, or death.

- Tachycardia, tachypnoea, hypotension, peripheral shut-down, haemodynamic collapse, raised JVP with a prominent 'a' wave, RV heave, gallop rhythm, widely-split second heart sound.
- Chest X-ray shows pulmonary oligaemia with prominence of main pulmonary trunk in hila.
- ECG shows sinus tachycardia, RA dilatation, RV strain, right axis deviation, new partial or complete RBBB; there may be AF, and T-wave inversion in right chest leads. S1 Q3 T3 pattern is rare.
- Pulmonary angiography or spiral CT may show PE.
- **Echo** shows a vigorous LV, dilated RA and RV, raised PASP assessed from TR if obstruction above the level of PV. PE may be seen in RVOT.

4. **Multiple recurrent PEs**. Gradual obstruction of regions of the pulmonary arterial circulation.
   - This may lead to progressive breathlessness over weeks or months due to gradual obstruction of regions of the pulmonary arterial circulation. May present non-specifically with weakness, angina, palpitations or exertional syncope.
   - On examination, there are physical signs of PHT due to multiple occlusions of the pulmonary vascular bed with signs of RV overload with an RV heave and loud P_2.
   - Chest X-ray may be normal.
   - V/Q scan shows multiple mismatched defects; leg and pelvic ultrasound may show abnormality.
   - **Echo** shows features of PHT with dilated RV and RA and raised PASP.

The echo findings in PE relate to the size of the embolism and the degree of obstruction of the pulmonary circulation. Important points are:

- A normal echo does not exclude PE (this is a particularly the case with small PEs).
- If there is pre-existing cardiovascular disease, this must be factored in to the echo findings.
- Massive PE. There is a right heart pressure and volume overload pattern with RV dilatation and possibly failure and RA dilatation.
- TR may occur due to increased right heart pressures.
- With medium-sized PE, there may be milder right heart dilatation and TR.
- LV assessment is essential. An inferior myocardial infarction with RV infarction may cause similar echo features of a dilated right heart, but there

will be normal PASP, unlike the situation with PE where the PASP will be raised.

- RV pressures rarely exceed 60–70 mmHg. If the pressure is over 70 mmHg in PE, the differential diagnosis includes acute on chronic PE or PE on the background of PHT.

Occasionally, it is possible to see that there is a PE in the proximal PA. Occasionally, a PE 'in transit' may be seen, either caught in the TV apparatus or sometimes intraoperatively during TOE. On contrast echo, a right-to-left shunt via PFO may be seen if the RA pressures increase and there may be bowing of the intra-atrial septum from right to left.

Echo features of a poorer prognosis with PE include:

- Significant right heart dilatation
- RV systolic dysfunction
- PE in transit.

Management of PE

- Acute treatment – resuscitation, high-concentration oxygen, analgesia, bedrest, fluids, inotropic support, intensive care
- Prevention of further PEs – anticoagulation (e.g. intravenous heparin then oral warfarin, usually for at least 6 months) or occasionally physical methods (e.g. insertion of a filter in the inferior vena cava above the level of the renal veins) if recurrent PEs or inability to take anticoagulants
- Dissolution of PE – thrombolytic therapy, e.g. intravenous streptokinase
- Surgery – removal of PE is rarely needed, if massive.

4.7 LONG-AXIS FUNCTION

Ventricular systole involves longitudinal (long-axis) as well as circumferential (short-axis) shortening. Long-axis function gives important information about normal cardiac physiology and disease states.

Echo assessment of long-axis function

The LV (Fig. 4.16) and RV long axes run from the apex (which is fixed relative to the chest wall) to the base of the heart (which is taken as the MV and TV rings). Function of separate parts can be examined (e.g. LV and RV free walls, IVS).

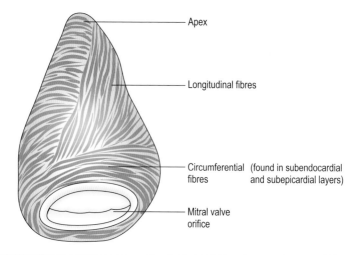

Fig. 4.16 *Schematic representation of the arrangement of fibres of left ventricle.*

Long-axis measurements are made using M-mode or Doppler echo. It is important to look at amplitude, velocity and timing of long-axis changes.

Long-axis contribution to normal physiology (Figs 4.17, 4.18)

1. Ejection fraction

Long-axis function plays a role in maintaining normal ejection fraction and changes in LV cavity shape.

2. Blood flow into atria

During ventricular systole, the MV and TV rings move towards the cardiac apex, increasing the capacity of the two atria as their floor moves downwards. Atrial volumes increase (and pressure falls), drawing blood into the atria from the caval and pulmonary veins.

3. Early diastolic flow

The MV moves backwards towards the LA during early diastolic forward blood flow into the LV. Effectively, blood that was in the LA finds itself in the LV as the MV ring has moved backwards around it. LV volume has increased without

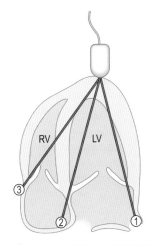

① **LV free (lateral) wall**
   – often supplied by circumflex artery
   ± left anterior descending

② **Interventricular septum**
   – left anterior descending artery

③ **RV free wall**
   – usually right coronary artery

Fig. 4.17 Long-axis function. M-mode study of movement of atrioventricular rings towards the apex.

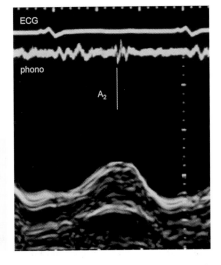

Fig. 4.18 Long-axis function. M-mode showing movement of the mitral valve ring (left ventricle free wall side) towards the apex during systole. An ECG and phonocardiogram are recorded to allow timing of events, such as aortic valve closure (A₂).

blood actually moving with respect to the apex and chest wall! This is not detectable on Doppler. This and a similar effect during atrial systole account for 10–15% of LV stroke volume and 20% of RV.

The LA is not a passive structure. During ventricular systole, the LA is subject to external work from the ventricle and this is transferred back to the LV during early diastole and coupled to blood flow.

4. Atrial systole

Atrial blood volume falls during atrial systole. The lateral and back walls of the atria are fixed to the mediastinum and the dominant mechanism by which their volume falls is by movement of the AV rings away from the ventricular apex.

Long-axis function in disease

1. Ventricular function

Long-axis function gives a good estimate of the EF of both ventricles. This is useful when an apical 4-chamber view can be taken and parasternal views are difficult, e.g. in a severely ill, ventilated patient on ITU.

Regional reduction in long-axis function is common after acute MI. These defects correlate with fixed defects on myocardial perfusion imaging (e.g. thallium).

After MV replacement, long-axis function is reduced, but not after MV repair or in MS. This does not occur consistently after cardiopulmonary bypass for other reasons and is likely to reflect loss of papillary muscle function.

In restrictive LV disease, long-axis amplitude is low even with a normal LV size at end-diastole.

2. Coronary artery disease and ischaemia

Long-axis function provides a remarkably sensitive, noninvasive assessment of ischaemia. This may be due to the fact that a significant proportion of longitudinal muscle fibres are located in the subendocardium. Long-axis function is often asynchronous in coronary disease (e.g. chronic stable angina) and segmental in distribution. Onset of contraction is often delayed. This effect may explain the 'abnormal relaxation' pattern of LV diastolic dysfunction seen with ageing (where the early E-wave on Doppler is reduced or absent and the A-wave increased).

3. Activation abnormalities

Long-axis function is sensitive to activation abnormalities possibly due to subendocardial location of fibres. Abnormalities occur in right bundle branch block (RBBB) and left bundle branch block (LBBB). This allows assessment of the effects of abnormal activation, especially in patients with severe ventricular disease and of different pacing modes in patients with heart failure.

4. LVH

LV diastolic function is abnormal in LVH even when short-axis systolic function is not. Long-axis function is often abnormal.

5. Atrial function

Restoration of atrial mechanical function after cardioversion of AF (section 7.2) can be demonstrated by long-axis function (RA is restored more rapidly than LA). Contraction of pectinate muscles causes movement of the atrioventricular ring. This is the earliest consequence of atrial mechanical activity.

4.8 PERICARDIAL DISEASE

The pericardium (Fig. 4.19) is the sac that surrounds the heart and is made up of the outer fibrous pericardium and the inner serous pericardium which has

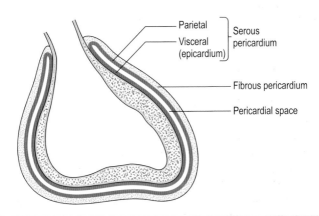

Fig. 4.19 *Layers of pericardium.*

an outer parietal layer (attached to the fibrous sac) and an inner visceral layer (or epicardium, attached to the heart).

There is a potential pericardial space between the 2 layers of serous pericardium normally containing a small volume (<50 mL) of pericardial fluid.

Echo is the most effective method to assess many of the pathological changes that may affect the pericardium causing an increase in pericardial fluid (pericardial effusion), cardiac tamponade or constrictive pericarditis. The normal fibrous pericardium is highly echo-reflective and appears echo-bright. Fluid in the pericardial space is poorly reflective and appears black.

1. Pericardial effusion

A pericardial effusion may be composed of serous fluid, blood or rarely pus (when the individual is very seriously ill).

Causes of pericardial effusion

- Infection – viral, bacterial including tuberculosis, fungal
- Malignancy
- Heart failure
- Post MI – Dressler's syndrome
- Cardiac trauma or surgery
- Uraemia
- Autoimmune – rheumatoid arthritis, SLE, scleroderma
- Inflammation – amyloid, sarcoid
- Hypothyroidism
- Drugs – phenylbutazone, penicillin, procainamide, hydralazine, isoniazid
- Aortic dissection
- Radiation
- Idiopathic.

M-mode and **2-D echo** are the most important methods to assess pericardial effusion (Figs 4.20, 4.21). On M-mode, using a parasternal long-axis view, the echo-free pericardial effusion may be seen below the posterior wall of the LV or above the anterior wall of the RV. On 2-D imaging, the effusion can be seen as an echo-free space surrounding the heart. The effusion may be throughout the pericardial space or loculated in certain regions only.

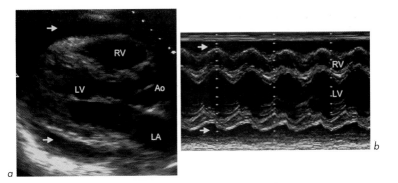

Fig. 4.20 *Pericardial effusion. **(a)** Parasternal long-axis view showing effusion anterior to right ventricle and posterior to left ventricle (arrows). **(b)** M-mode showing effusion (arrows).*

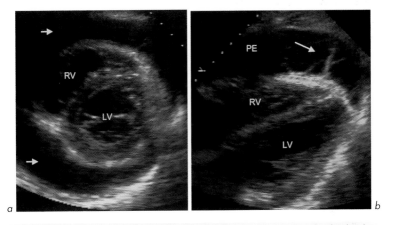

Fig. 4.21 *Pericardial effusion. **(a)** Parasternal short-axis view at mitral valve level showing effusion (arrows). **(b)** Magnified subcostal view showing fibrin strands (arrow) in the effusion (PE).*

Differentiation between pericardial and pleural effusion can be made on 2-D or M-mode (although the 2 may co-exist) (Fig. 4.22). Unlike pleural effusion, the echo-free space of pericardial effusion terminates at the AV groove and does not extend beyond the level of the descending aorta.

109

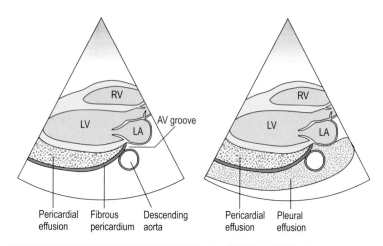

Fig. 4.22 *Differentiation between pericardial effusion and pleural effusion on 2-D echo.*

Estimation of the volume of pericardial effusion present can be made by echo. This can be done qualitatively on M-mode or 2-D by the depth to the echo-free space around the heart. A more accurate method is to use the planimetry (area estimation) function present on most echo machine computers. A still image of an apical 4-chamber view is taken and the following measurements made:

1. A tracing around the pericardium (from which the computer calculates the combined volumes of the heart and pericardium)
2. A tracing around the heart (which gives the volume of the heart).

The volume of the effusion is obtained by subtracting these volumes.

2. Cardiac tamponade

This is a dangerous situation in which cardiac function is impaired due to external pressure upon the heart, e.g. due to fluid accumulation or pericardial constriction. Tamponade may result from a large volume of pericardial effusion or a rapidly forming small volume of effusion which causes pressure on the heart (very large effusions can form without causing tamponade if the pericardial sac has time to stretch to accommodate the fluid).

Clinical features of tamponade

- Tachycardia (heart rate >100)
- Hypotension (systolic BP <100 mmHg) with a small pulse volume
- Pulsus paradoxus of >10 mmHg (an exaggeration of the normal small – <5 mmHg – fall in systolic BP during inspiration)
- Raised JVP with a prominent 'X' systolic descent. The JVP may not fall as normal on inspiration or infrequently may paradoxically rise (Kussmaul's paradox).

Remember: Tamponade is a **clinical** diagnosis. Echo can provide supportive evidence of it.

Echo features of tamponade

- Large volume pericardial effusion.
- RA and/or RV diastolic collapse. Both are sensitive to tamponade. After relief of tamponade by drainage of the effusion, RV diastolic collapse soon reverses. Diastolic RA collapse does not do so as quickly and may be the more sensitive indicator of tamponade.
- Doppler features are of exaggerated changes in transmitral and transtricuspid flows normally seen with inspiration and expiration and changes in flow patterns of the superior vena cava (SVC).

Echo may aid in safely performing therapeutic echo-guided needle aspiration of pericardial fluid (pericardiocentesis) to relieve the tamponade, which may be life saving. Echo can help to locate the site and extent of fluid collection and assess the success of the procedure.

3. Acute pericarditis

This is inflammation of the pericardium and has a number of causes. There may be associated pericardial effusion. The clinical features vary widely. Some individuals may be relatively asymptomatic, while others suffer a severe illness with inflammation extending to the myocardium (myopericarditis) with haemodynamic collapse. Acute pericarditis may be recurrent.

Clinical features of acute pericarditis

- Chest pain which is retrosternal and may be referred to the shoulders or neck. The pain is worsened by respiration, usually by taking a deep breath (pleuritic chest pain) and by movement. The pain is often worse on lying flat and improved by sitting forward.

- Fever, especially when pericarditis is due to viral or bacterial infection, myocardial infarction or rheumatic fever.
- Malaise.
- Pericardial friction rub. This is a scratching/crunching superficial sound. It has been described as the sound made by the feet when 'walking on snow'.

Causes of pericarditis

- Idiopathic
- Viral infection – e.g. Coxsackie
- Myocardial infarction – acute or 1 month to 1 year later (Dressler's syndrome)
- Uraemia – in the terminal stages of renal failure and may be asymptomatic
- Malignancy – especially carcinoma of bronchus or breast, Hodgkin's lymphoma, leukaemia, malignant melanoma
- Tuberculosis – low-grade fever (especially in the evening) with malaise, weight loss and features of acute pericarditis (pericardial aspiration may be needed to diagnose)
- Bacterial – purulent pericarditis with pneumonia, e.g. *Staphylococcus aureus*, *Haemophilus influenzae*, or septicaemia; often fatal; treatment is with antibiotics with or without surgical drainage
- Trauma
- Radiotherapy – only if the heart is not fully shielded.

Investigations

The ECG is diagnostic showing ST elevation with a saddle-shaped concave upwards ST segment (Fig. 4.23). The inflammatory markers (ESR and C-reactive protein) and white blood cell count are elevated. Cardiac enzymes and troponins may be elevated if there is associated myocarditis.

Treatment

Non-steroidal anti-inflammatory drugs and steroids are given if the pericarditis is severe or recurrent.

An **echo** is often requested for individuals who clinically have acute pericarditis.

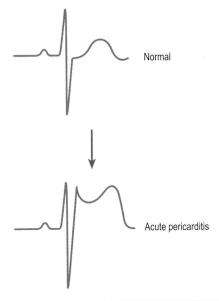

Fig. 4.23 *ECG in acute pericarditis showing 'saddle-shaped' ST segment elevation (arrow).*

Echo features of acute pericarditis

- The echo may be normal with no pathognomonic features in uncomplicated viral pericarditis
- There may be a pericardial effusion
- Associated features, e.g. regional wall motion abnormalities with acute myocardial infarction
- 'Thickened' pericardium.

Use of echo in acute pericarditis

- Aids in diagnosis of underlying aetiology
- Detects complications such as effusion, myopericarditis, systolic and diastolic ventricular dysfunction
- Associated pericardial effusion

- Regional wall motion abnormalities
- Tumour detection
- Differential diagnosis from conditions with similar presentation, e.g. vegetations and MR in a patient with fever, systolic murmur or rub due to infective endocarditis
- In subjects with chest pain within 12 hours of an acute coronary syndrome to differentiate myocardial damage (wall motion abnormalities) from pericarditis.

4. Constrictive pericarditis

In this condition, the fibrous pericardium becomes more rigid and often calcifies, limiting the diastolic expansion of the ventricles and reducing diastolic filling.

Causes of constrictive pericarditis
- Tuberculosis
- Connective tissue disorders
- Malignancy
- Trauma and post-cardiac surgery
- Uraemia
- Other infection – bacterial, viral
- Idiopathic.

It can be difficult to diagnose this accurately on echo, and it is particularly hard to distinguish from restrictive cardiomyopathy or a restrictive myocardial function pattern due to myocardial infiltration. Direct pressure measurements at catheterization studies may be needed to make the diagnosis.

Echo features of constrictive pericarditis
M-mode and 2-D echo
- Thickened pericardium. This is difficult to quantify and often tends to be overestimated. The normal pericardium is highly echogenic and appears bright. The degree of this depends upon the gain settings on the echo machine. On M-mode, the thickened pericardium appears as a dark thick echo line or as multiple separated parallel lines.

- Calcified pericardium – localized or generalized.
- Abnormal septal motion, especially end-diastolic (exaggerated anterior motion).
- Dilated IVC due to raised systemic venous pressure.
- Abnormal LV filling pattern – LV only expands in early diastole. Difficult to recognize in real-time. On M-mode this appears as mid- and late-diastolic flattening of LVPW motion.
- Premature diastolic opening of the PV with increased RV end-diastolic pressure.

Doppler

Abnormal MV flow pattern reflecting abnormal diastolic LV filling of a 'restrictive pattern'.

- Increase in early diastolic velocity (E-wave large)
- Rapid deceleration
- Very small A-wave compared with E
- Short pressure half-time of mitral and tricuspid valve flow
- Exaggerated respiratory variation of MV flow (decreased E-wave by >25% on inspiration) or TV flow (decreased E-wave by >25% on expiration).

There is also prominent systolic 'X' descent of SVC flow.

4.9 DEVICE THERAPY FOR HEART FAILURE – CARDIAC RESYNCHRONIZATION THERAPY

There have been recent advances in the management of heart failure. Implantable electrical device therapy has become an option for some patients. Patients with heart failure may have poor coordination of the electrical activation and of the systolic and diastolic function of the LV and RV (known as *mechanical dyssynchrony*). They may have other problems affecting cardiac output, such as MR. Cardiac resynchronization therapy (CRT) is a technique of simultaneous biventricular pacing which aims to improve the haemodynamic situation. CRT has added to the treatment options for patients, especially those with severe, drug-refractory and drug-optimized heart failure. CRT is not suitable for all individuals with heart failure, so methods have to be devised to select potential responders. Echo plays an important part in the selection of patients and in optimizing therapy and monitoring progress.

How is CRT carried out?

CRT involves the implantation in the upper chest of an electrical pulse generator (pacemaker) device from which three pacing leads descend via veins into the heart (Figs 4.24 and 4.25). Leads are placed into the RA, RV and LV (the latter usually via the coronary sinus). These CRT pacing (CRT-P) devices are used to improve cardiac function by resynchronizing atrial, RV and LV function. Some devices also include a cardiovertor-defibrillator function (these are known as CRT-D devices) and evidence suggests that these devices reduce mortality from VT and VF. Some devices also allow an estimation of thoracic impedance with changes in the degree of pulmonary interstitial fluid, which may give the patient or doctor an early indication of the development of pulmonary oedema.

Echo can be used to assess ventricular systolic and diastolic function (e.g. LVEF) and look for evidence of dyssynchrony and other features in heart failure, such as MR.

Abnormal electrical activation and mechanical dyssynchrony in heart failure

The QRS complex of the ECG represents the vector sum of the electrical forces within the ventricular myocardium with time. Normal electrical activity

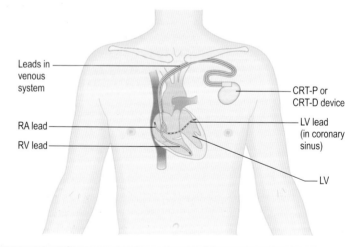

Leads in venous system

CRT-P or CRT-D device

RA lead

LV lead (in coronary sinus)

RV lead

LV

Fig. 4.24 *Cardiac resynchronization therapy (CRT) using a pacemaker (CRT-P) or a defibrillator (CRT-D).*

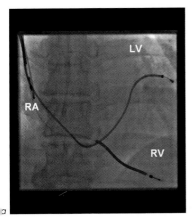
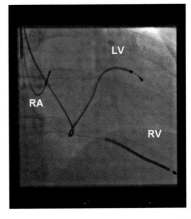

Fig. 4.25 *Chest radiographs showing 3 CRT leads in the heart. (a) Antero-posterior and (b) right anterior oblique projections. The LV lead is in the coronary sinus.*

propagates through the myocardial Purkinje network (Fig. 4.26). In damaged myocardium, conduction is impaired, changing the velocity and direction of electrical propagation and causing abnormal electrical activity. Abnormal ventricular depolarization generates regions of delayed and early ventricular contraction causing dyssynchronized mechanical activity and impairing systolic and diastolic function.

In heart failure, there may be:

- Interventricular dyssynchrony – poor coordination of activation of LV relative to RV
- Intraventricular dyssynchrony – delayed activation of one LV region relative to another.

Abnormal depolarization is manifest on the ECG as QRS prolongation (bundle branch block, BBB). The pattern may be of left (LBBB), right (RBBB) or non-specific intraventricular conduction delay. The normal QRS duration is under 120 ms. There is a direct relationship between QRS duration and ejection fraction and some have demonstrated a good correlation between QRS duration and interventricular mechanical dyssynchrony. RBBB may be a normal finding

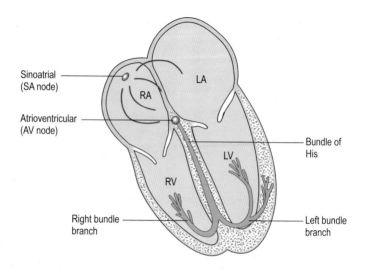

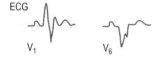

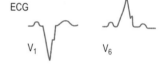

Causes of RBBB

- normal variant in 1–5% of population
- idiopathic conducting tissue disease/fibrosis
- congenital heart disease – ASD, VSD, PS, tetralogy of Fallot
- myocardial disease – cardiomyopathy
- coronary artery disease – acute MI
- pulmonary disease – cor pulmonale
- recurrent multiple PEs
- acute PE
- drugs and electrolyte abnormalities – class IA drugs, hypokalaemia
- RV surgery.

Causes of LBBB

- idiopathic conducting tissue disease/fibrosis
- myocardial disease – cardiomyopathy
- coronary artery disease – acute MI, severe multi-vessel disease
- LVOT – AS
- LVH – hypertension

Fig. 4.26 *Myocardial conduction system – Purkinje network.*

in up to 5% of the population. LBBB is pathological. Bundle branch block occurs in about 20% of the heart failure population, but in over 35% of patients with severe heart failure, and bundle branch block is a strong independent predictor of mortality.

QRS duration, especially with LBBB pattern, was initially used as the main selection criterion for CRT. Those with QRS durations >150 ms are more likely to respond than those with QRS durations of 120–150 ms. A beneficial response to CRT was initially considered to result in part from resynchronization of interventricular dyssynchrony (dyssynchrony between LV and RV). QRS duration alone, however, is a poor predictor of response to CRT and 20–30% of patients fail to respond to CRT despite prolonged QRS duration. It has subsequently been suggested that LV dyssynchrony may predict response to CRT more accurately than interventricular dyssynchrony. While data indicate that patients with a wider QRS complex have a higher likelihood of LV dyssynchrony, over 30% of patients with wide QRS lack LV dyssynchrony. This 30% may partially explain a similar percentage of non-responders in the studies. These observations have resulted in many echo studies evaluating different echo parameters to detect LV dyssynchrony and predict response to CRT.

Echo techniques have thus been developed to assess mechanical dyssynchrony with the aim of identifying potential responders to CRT. Echo can also measure LVEF and assess severity of MR in heart failure.

Aims of CRT

- Resynchronization of intraventricular contraction
- Resynchronization of interventricular contraction
- Optimization of atrioventricular coordination
- Reduction in MR
- Haemodynamic improvement
- Reversal of maladaptive remodelling of the ventricles
- Improvement in symptoms
- Improvement in prognosis.

Studies suggest that in correctly selected individuals with heart failure, CRT can lead to:
- Improved functional status
- Reduced hospitalization
- Improved symptoms

- Improved quality of life
- Increased exercise capacity
- Reduced mortality.

CRT also improves echo endpoints including:
- Improved LV systolic function
- Reduced LV size and volumes
- Reduced MR
- LV 'reverse remodelling' as indicated by decreased systolic and diastolic diameters and volumes.

Uses of echo in CRT

1. Patient selection – identifying potential responders to treatment
2. Optimization of CRT following device implantation
3. Monitoring and assessing progress and outcome.

1. Patient selection for CRT

Some clinical studies have based selection of patients for CRT upon ECG criteria, but evidence suggests a beneficial role for echo. Echo may be of help in CRT in the selection of patients and the prediction of who may respond to treatment and those who can avoid an unnecessary procedure (i.e. narrow QRS responders and wide QRS non-responders). Some studies suggest 20–30% of these patients are non-responders and propose that echo assessment may be more beneficial by determining mechanical dyssynchrony.

Echo assessment of mechanical dyssynchrony – interventricular and LV dyssynchrony

Echo is the most practical approach to evaluate mechanical dyssynchrony and predict response to CRT. A number of echo techniques are used to identify potential responders to CRT. These include conventional M-mode, 2-D echo and Doppler techniques with tissue Doppler imaging (TDI) and newer techniques, including 3-D echo, some of which are complex and require considerable postprocessing and analysis.

TDI is the most extensively used technique and different methods have been proposed including pulsed wave TDI, colour-coded TDI, tissue tracking, displacement mapping, strain and strain rate imaging, and tissue synchronization imaging (TSI).

Echo can be used to examine both interventricular and LV intraventricular dyssynchrony. None of the techniques is ideal, and they should be used in combination. There is limited evidence of the usefulness of individual echo techniques to predict response to CRT. No single parameter should be used to decide implantation. Initial studies focused on assessment of interventricular (LV to RV) dyssynchrony to predict response but most studies suggest that *LV intraventricular dyssynchrony is a more useful predictor of response to CRT than interventricular dyssynchrony* and some reports suggest that interventricular dyssynchrony is not related to haemodynamic improvement after CRT.

Other factors which may influence the response to CRT include:

- Coronary venous anatomy – impacts upon LV lead placement and can be assessed by venography (Fig. 4.27)
- Presence of scar tissue – affects lead placement and can be assessed by echo, MRI and nuclear medicine techniques such as technetium-99 m labelling.

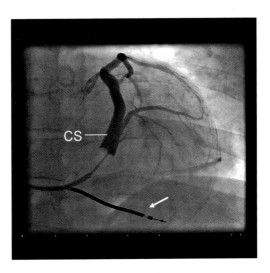

Fig. 4.27 *Coronary venogram prior to insertion of coronary sinus (CS) lead for CRT. The RV lead is shown (arrow).*

Echo techniques to assess mechanical dyssynchrony

M-mode

- Parasternal long axis septal to posterior wall motion delay of over 130 ms is a marker of LV dyssynchrony.

2-D echo

- A semi-automated method can be used for endocardial border detection. Apical four-chamber views to look at the septal-to-lateral wall relationship can be used to generate wall motion curves. Echo contrast techniques can be used to optimize LV border detection to determine dyssynchrony between septum and lateral walls and assess the degree of LV dyssynchrony. Computer-generated regional wall motion movement curves are compared by mathematical trace analysis based on Fourier transformation to give a measure of LV dyssynchrony. With improved LV border detection, regional and fractional area changes are determined and plotted versus time, yielding displacement maps. From these maps, the LV dyssynchrony between the septum and lateral wall is determined. Using this approach, some patients with extensive LV dyssynchrony between the septum and lateral wall exhibit an immediate improvement in haemodynamics with CRT.

Pulsed wave and continuous wave Doppler

- These can be used to evaluate the extent of interventricular mechanical delay defined as a time difference between LV and RV pre-ejection intervals. A delay of >40 ms has been proposed as a marker of interventricular dyssynchrony.
- Flow across the LVOT and RVOT. This can determine the time of onset of flow across the AV and PV. With simultaneous recording of the ECG, it is possible to determine the delay between the onset of the QRS and the onset of flow. This gives the aortic and pulmonary pre-ejection periods (A-PEP and P-PEP), markers of electro-mechanical delay (EMD). The normal A-PEP is under 140 ms but an increase in A-PEP on its own as a marker of LV dyssynchrony is probably not a useful predictor for CRT. The interventricular mechanical delay (A-PEP minus P-PEP) is usually under 40 ms. This measure may be more helpful in CRT assessment.
- The transmitral pulsed wave Doppler can be used to measure the diastolic filling time (the time from the onset of the mitral E-wave to the end of the

A-wave) as a percentage of the cardiac cycle length. The normal value is over 40%. Alone, this is probably not a useful measure for predicting CRT response, but may be useful at baseline and at CRT follow-up.

Tissue Doppler imaging (TDI)

TDI techniques are probably the most used to assess dyssynchrony.

- **Pulsed wave TDI**, using 2-, 4- or 12-segment models of LV dyssynchrony, is used to predict response to CRT. TDI measures the velocity of longitudinal cardiac motion and allows comparison of timing of wall motion in relation to electrical activity (QRS complex). The delay between the QRS and the onset of mechanical activity is the electro-mechanical delay (EMD). Different parameters are derived, e.g. peak systolic velocity, time to onset of systolic velocity, time to peak systolic velocity. These can be obtained directly using pulsed wave TDI but this method allows only one area to be examined at a time and therefore is time-consuming and cannot compare segments simultaneously. Measurements are influenced by differences in heart rate, load conditions and respiration. In addition, the timing of peak systolic velocity is often difficult to identify, resulting in imprecise information on LV dyssynchrony. This method is not able to differentiate between active or passive movement of myocardial segments. TDI has also been used to assess interventricular dyssynchrony by comparing the delay between peak systolic velocity of the RV and LV free walls.
- **Colour-coded TDI** can be used to assess LV dyssynchrony. From these colour-coded images, which need post-processing, TDI tracings can be obtained and used to show the time to peak systolic velocity in order to assess LV dyssynchrony. Initially, investigators focused on the 4-chamber view to identify LV dyssynchrony by colour-coded TDI. Velocity tracings are derived from the basal, septal and lateral segments and the septal to lateral delay was measured. It was shown that a delay of over 60 ms was predictive of acute response to CRT. Subsequently, a 4-segment model was applied which included 4 basal segments (septal, lateral, inferior and anterior). A delay of over 65 ms allows prediction of response to CRT.

Other TDI techniques have been devised, the details of which are beyond the scope of this book; they include:

- **Tissue tracking.** This is calculated as the integral of the velocity curve with time and shows the displacement of tissue during the cycle. It does not

123

distinguish between active and passive movement of a myocardial segment. It provides a colour-coded display of myocardial displacement, allowing for easy visualization of LV dyssynchrony and the region of latest activation.

- **Strain rate.** Calculated as dv/ds (dv is the difference in velocities between adjacent measuring points and ds is the distance between these points). It shows velocity of deformation as rate/s. Timing of cardiac events during the cardiac cycle can be measured more accurately than with other TDI methods. A disadvantage is that it is angle-dependent and easily influenced by noise.

- **Strain analysis** (integral of strain rate over time) can help to distinguish active from passive movement but it is angle-dependent and influenced by noise.

  Strain rate and strain analysis are performed by offline analysis of the colour-coded tissue Doppler images. Strain analysis allows direct assessment of the extent of myocardial deformation, with time, during systole and is expressed as the percentage of segmental shortening or lengthening in relation to its original length. The main advantage over TDI is that strain analysis allows differentiation between active systolic contraction and passive motion of segments. This is important in patients with ischaemic cardiomyopathy in the presence of scar tissue.

- **Tissue synchronization imaging (TSI).** TSI is a signal processing algorithm of the tissue Doppler data to detect automatically the peak myocardial velocity and then colour code these. It is a recent addition to TDI approaches to assessing LV dyssynchrony. The automated colour coding of time to reach peak longitudinal velocities can be superimposed on 2-D echo images to provide visual and mechanical information on the anatomical region. LV dyssynchrony can be defined as the difference in times to peak velocity of opposing walls – inferoseptal to lateral wall (4-chamber view), anterior to inferior wall (2-chamber view) and anteroseptal to posterior wall (long-axis view). Recent technical advances include multi-plane TSI imaging with 3-D reconstruction of colour-coded temporal LV activation.

3-D echo in CRT

3-D echo can be used to:

- Assess LV volumes and LVEF.
- Examine regional wall motion abnormalities. This gives an indication of LV dyssynchrony (analysis of regional function) and the degree of dispersion of segmental volume changes. The change in volume for each segment (using 16 or 17 segments models of LV) throughout the cycle can be shown. With

synchronous contraction of all segments, each segment is expected to achieve its minimum volume at almost the same point of the cardiac cycle. In LV dyssynchrony, dispersion exists in the timing of the point of minimum volume for each segment. The degree of dispersion reflects the severity of LV dyssynchrony.

- Quantify valvular regurgitation (e.g. MR).
- Guide electrophysiologists in selecting optimum lead placement positions by using parametric 'polar map' displays of the 3-D data of the timing of LV contraction.

Currently, no extensive data are available on the prediction of response to CRT using 3-D echo.

2. Optimization of CRT following device implantation

Echo also plays a role in the optimization of pacemaker settings after CRT. Changes in atrioventricular and interventricular pacing delays can improve benefit from CRT (Fig. 4.28). The response to CRT leads to some immediate benefits (acute improvement in haemodynamic parameters such as cardiac output and improvements in MR) and long-term benefits (improvement in clinical parameters, systolic LV function, reverse LV remodelling and further reduction in MR).

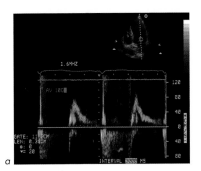
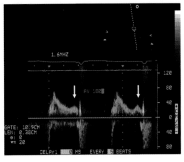

a b

Fig. 4.28 *CRT optimization. Pulsed wave Doppler at LV inflow. Changing the atrioventricular time interval from (a) 100 ms to (b) 180 ms, by altering the pacemaker settings, improves LV filling with the emergence of an A-wave (arrows).*

125

Optimization of atrioventricular and interventricular (VV) delays in CRT

Optimization of these pacemaker settings may further enhance benefit from CRT. Both atrioventricular and VV delays can be optimized using modern CRT devices. Doppler echo can be used to optimize atrioventricular delay (Fig. 4.28). This echo-guided optimization appears crucial in some heart failure patients, who may exhibit an acute increase in cardiac output of up to 50%. It is carried out by determining the optimum atrioventricular delay to allow the end of the Doppler A-wave, corresponding to LA contraction, to occur just before the onset of aortic systolic Doppler flow. The effects of optimization can also be examined by looking at the reduction in LV dyssynchrony and increases in LVEF.

Reduction in MR

Reduction in MR has been reported after CRT and can be improved by VV optimization. The severity of MR can be examined by echo Doppler techniques.

3. Who is a responder to CRT?

Use of echo to monitor and assess long-term progress and outcome of CRT

Despite acute improvements with CRT, deciding who is a long-term responder to CRT can be difficult to assess objectively and to quantify. There is a placebo effect with CRT in about 40% of patients.

Small studies initially used invasive methods to assess acute haemodynamic response to CRT. Long-term response is usually assessed at 3 to 6 months of CRT. It is mainly evaluated by clinical or echo parameters. The relationship between acute haemodynamic response and chronic outcomes is still not entirely clear.

In patients who improve clinically following CRT, clinical and echo response may not occur simultaneously. Some patients who show clinical improvement may not exhibit improved echo parameters, such as reverse remodelling (which can be defined as >15% reduction in LV end-systolic volume) and vice versa. More patients exhibit improved clinical parameters than improved echo markers. This discrepancy further complicates the initial selection of patients.

CRT leads to changes in LV size, LV volumes, LVEF, and reverse remodelling (indicated by decreases in LV systolic and diastolic diameters and volumes, Fig. 4.29), and improves LV and interventricular dyssynchrony. Echo can help to measure these changes. The ultimate clinical endpoints include a reduction in hospitalization and mortality rates.

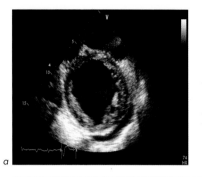
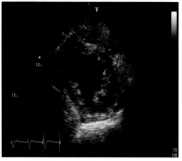

a   b

Fig. 4.29 *Reverse remodelling following CRT. Parasternal short-axis views showing LV at end-diastole at* **(a)** *baseline and* **(b)** *6 months following implantation of CRT device.*

Markers of long-term response to CRT

Clinical
- NYHA functional class
- Quality-of-life score
- 6-minute walk distance
- Peak VO$_2$ exercise capacity
- Heart failure hospitalizations
- Cardiac mortality

Echo
- LVEF
- LV dimensions/volumes
- Reverse remodelling
- MR
- Interventricular resynchronization
- LV resynchronization

Adapted from Bax et al *J Am Coll Cardiol* 2005; 46:2168–2182.

Guidelines

Guidelines have been prepared suggesting which patients with heart failure may benefit from CRT (see below).

Indications for CRT

Cardiac resynchronization therapy with a pacing device (CRT-P) is recommended as a treatment option for people with heart failure who fulfil *all* the following criteria (adapted from NICE Technology Guidance Appraisal 120, May 2007):

1. They are currently experiencing or have recently experienced NYHA class III–IV symptoms.
2. They are in sinus rhythm either with a QRS duration of 150 ms or longer estimated by standard ECG or with a QRS duration of 120–149 ms estimated by ECG and mechanical dyssynchrony that is confirmed by echocardiography.
3. They have LVEF of 35% or less.
4. They are receiving optimal pharmacological therapy.

Cardiac resynchronization therapy with a defibrillator device (CRT-D) may be considered for people who fulfil the criteria for implantation of a CRT-P device, but who also separately fulfil the criteria for the use of an ICD device (adapted from NICE Technology Guidance Appraisal 95, 2006):

Secondary prevention for patients who present in the absence of a treatable cause with one of the following:

1. Having survived a cardiac arrest due to either VT or VF
2. Spontaneous sustained VT causing syncope or significant haemodynamic compromise
3. Sustained VT without syncope or cardiac arrest, and who have an associated LVEF of less than 35% (no worse than class III of New York Heart Association functional classification).

Primary prevention for patients who have one of the following:

1. A history of previous (more than 4 weeks) myocardial infarction and
   either
   LV dysfunction with LVEF of less than 35% (no worse than class III of New York Heart Association classification) and non-sustained VT on Holter 24-hour ECG monitoring and inducible VT on electrophysiological studies
   or
   LV dysfunction with LVEF of less than 30% and QRS duration of equal or more than 120 ms.
2. A familial cardiac condition with a high risk of sudden death, including long QT syndrome, hypertrophic cardiomyopathy, Brugada syndrome or arrhythmogenic right ventricular dysplasia (ARVD), or who have undergone surgical repair of congenital heart disease. ICDs may be used in other patient groups, for example those with dilated cardiomyopathy.

CHAPTER 5

Transoesophageal and stress echo and other echo techniques

5.1 TRANSOESOPHAGEAL ECHO

The echo techniques described so far have used ultrasound directed from the chest wall – transthoracic echo (TTE). The oesophagus in its mid-course lies posterior to and very close to the heart and ascending aorta and anterior to the descending aorta (Fig. 5.1).

An echo technique exists for examining the heart with a transducer in the oesophagus – transoesophageal echo (TOE) (Figs 5.2, 5.3, 5.4, 5.5). In some countries, the abbreviation used is TEE. This uses a transducer mounted upon a modified probe similar to those used for upper gastrointestinal endoscopy and allows examination of the heart without the barrier to ultrasound usually provided by the ribs, chest wall and lungs. By advancing the probe tip to various depths in the oesophagus and stomach, manoeuvring the tip of the transducer and by altering the angle of the ultrasound beam with controls placed on the handle, a number of different views of the heart can be obtained.

Advantages of TOE

- Improved image quality and resolution – the transducer is very close to the heart and there is less interference with the ultrasound beam. Higher ultrasound frequencies can be used since tissue attenuation of ultrasound is small and penetration depth required less than TTE (e.g. 5 MHz rather than 2–4 MHz).
- Some aspects of the heart can be examined which cannot be seen by TTE, e.g. posterior parts such as LA appendage, descending aorta, and pulmonary veins.

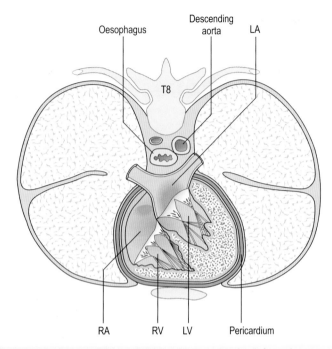

Fig. 5.1 *Cross-section of thorax at 8th thoracic vertebra level (from above).*

Disadvantages of TOE

- Invasive technique – uncomfortable with potential small risk
- New views have to be learnt.

Because of the invasive nature of TOE, it should only be performed if there is a good indication and after TTE has been performed. TOE-derived information should be used to complement that derived from TTE and not as an alternative. The potential risks of TOE (e.g. oesophageal damage) should be weighed up carefully against the potential benefits.

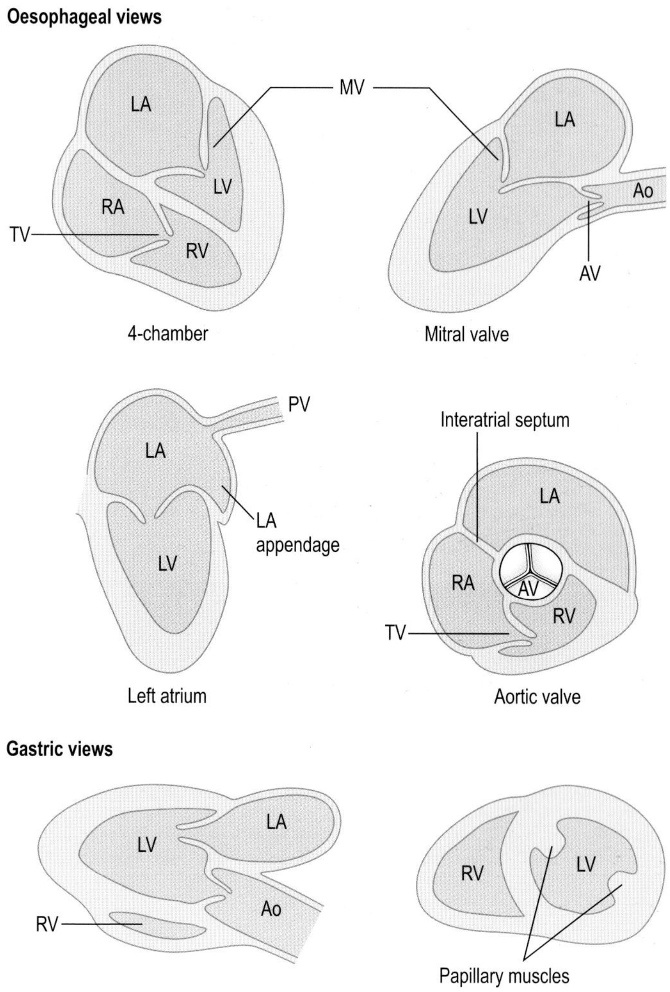

Fig. 5.2 Standard TOE views.

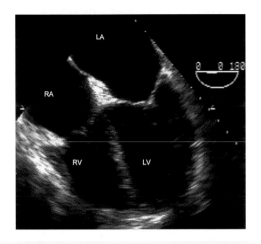

Fig. 5.3 4-chamber view using TOE.

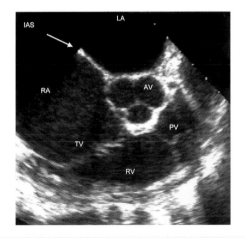

Fig. 5.4 Structures at aortic valve level on short-axis view using TOE. The interatrial septum is shown (arrow).

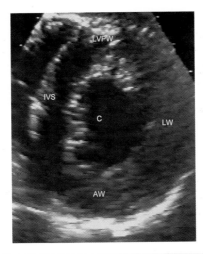

Fig. 5.5 *Short-axis view of left ventricle using TOE – transgastric view. AW, anterior wall; C, cavity; IVS, interventricular septum; LVPW, left ventricular posterior wall; LW, lateral wall.*

Uses of TOE

- **Mitral valve disease** – stenosis (anatomy of valve and subvalvular apparatus and assessment of suitability for valve repair rather than replacement or for balloon mitral valvotomy); prolapse (suitability for repair); regurgitation (severity and suitability for repair)
- **Endocarditis** – vegetations; abscess
- **Prosthetic valves** – haemodynamics; stability; endocarditis
- **Aortic disease** – dissection of ascending, arch or descending thoracic aorta; trauma; atheroma
- **Aortic valve disease**
- **Thromboembolic vascular disease** – stroke/TIA or peripheral embolism
- **Left atrial appendage** – thrombus
- **Intracardiac masses** – myxoma or other tumour; thrombus
- **Septal defects** – atrial (especially assessment for suitability for percutaneous closure); ventricular; contrast studies
- **Intraoperative monitoring** – assessment of mitral valve repair; left ventricular function and regional wall motion abnormalities; myomectomy

- **Congenital heart disease** – anatomy; haemodynamic assessment
- **Critically ill individuals on ITU**
- **Air or fat embolism** – haemodynamics.

Patient preparation and care during TOE

The patient should give informed consent being aware of the potential risks which include:

- Oesophageal trauma or perforation
- The risks of intravenous sedation
- Aspiration of stomach contents into lungs.

The patient should have fasted for at least 4 h. All false and loose teeth should be removed. There should be no history of difficulty in swallowing solids or liquids (dysphagia) which might suggest oesophageal disease. It is advisable to give oxygen during the procedure via nasal cannulae, to monitor blood oxygen with a pulse oximeter and to have suction equipment available to remove saliva from the mouth. Continuous ECG monitoring should be carried out as with any echo examination. Resuscitation equipment should be available.

A local anaesthetic spray (e.g. lidocaine (lignocaine) 10%) is used on the pharynx. Several sprays are given and there may be some systemic absorption. Intravenous sedation with a short-acting agent such as the benzodiazepine midazolam is often used. The patient is placed in the left lateral position with the neck fully flexed to aid insertion of the transducer into the oesophagus. A plastic bite guard is placed in the mouth to protect the transducer and the fingers of the person performing the TOE.

It is unusual to need to give a general anaesthetic (e.g. if TOE is considered essential and the patient is unable to tolerate the procedure under local anaesthesia and i.v. sedation). TOE is often carried out as a day-case procedure. After the procedure, the patient should not eat or drink for at least 1 hour (to prevent aspiration into the lungs or burning of the throat) since the throat remains numb and the patient may still be drowsy.

Contraindications to TOE

- Inability or refusal of the patient to give informed consent
- Dysphagia of unknown cause

- Oesophageal disease – tumour, oesophagitis, oesophageal varices, diverticulum, stricture, Mallory–Weiss tear, tracheo-oesophageal fistula
- Severe cervical arthritis or instability
- Bleeding gastric ulcer
- Severe pulmonary disease with hypoxaemia.

Complications of TOE (0.2–0.5%)

- Trauma – ranges from minor bleeding to oesophageal perforation
- Hypoxia
- Arrhythmia – SVT, AF, VT
- Laryngospasm or bronchospasm
- Angina
- Drug-related – respiratory depression, allergic reaction.

Specific uses of TOE

1. Cardiac or aortic source of embolism

TOE is often carried out in young patients (age <50 years) who have had a stroke. Approximately 20% may have a cardiac embolic source.

Detection of intracardiac thrombus with TTE is difficult with a high false-negative rate despite high suspicion on clinical grounds. TOE is superior not only because of improved image resolution but also because it is better at viewing areas where thrombus is likely to occur, such as LA appendage. This is the commonest site for thrombus, usually in patients with underlying heart disease.

Risk factors for LA thrombus include:
- MV disease (especially MS)
- AF
- LA dilatation
- Low-output states (e.g. heart failure).

In some studies of patients with cerebral ischaemia (TIA and stroke), up to 5% had LA thrombus and in 75% of cases this was in the LA appendage (Fig. 5.6). Thrombus may appear as a rounded or ovoid mass that may completely fill the appendage. False-positive diagnosis of thrombus may occur due to misinterpretation of LA anatomy:

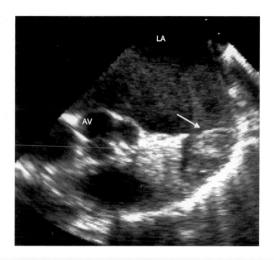

Fig. 5.6 *Thrombus in left atrial appendage (arrow). There is also spontaneous echo contrast in the left atrial cavity.*

1. Trabeculation of LA may be misdiagnosed as small thrombi
2. The ridge between the LA appendage and left upper pulmonary vein may be misdiagnosed as thrombus.

Spontaneous echo contrast

A swirling 'smoke-like' pattern of echo densities within any cardiac chamber is known as spontaneous contrast. It is usually seen in low-output states. It is most often seen in the LA in mitral disease (up to one-third of cases), especially MS where it may occur in up to 50% of cases. It is due to sluggish flow and is associated with clumping of red cells (rouleaux formation) which become more echo-reflective. There is an increased thromboembolic risk – LA thrombus occurs in 20–30% of those with spontaneous contrast.

Other LA structural abnormalities associated with increased thromboembolic risk include ASD, patent foramen ovale (PFO) and atrial septal aneurysm.

Atrial septal aneurysm (Fig. 5.7)

This is a bulging of the fossa ovalis and is found at autopsy in 1% of individuals. For echo purposes, the bulge must involve 1.5 cm of the septum and protrude

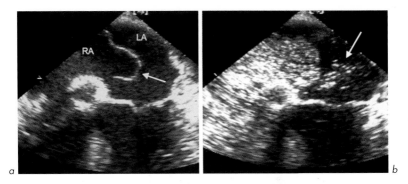

Fig. 5.7 *Atrial septal aneurysm on TOE study. (a) Aneurysm bulging into left atrium (arrow). There appears to be a defect at lower region of aneurysm, probably a patent foramen ovale. (b) Bubble contrast study showing bubbles crossing from right to left atrium (arrow) through an associated patent foramen ovale.*

1.1 cm into either atrium. It is found in 0.2% of TTE series. In suspected cardiac source of embolism, it occurs in up to 15% of cases. The association with TIA/stroke may be because the aneurysm is thrombogenic and/or due to its frequent association with PFO and ASDs, which may allow paradoxical right to left embolization. TOE can help to detect all of these. A bubble contrast study during TOE can help to identify a small ASD or PFO and show a small shunt (section 6.4).

TOE can show thrombus in other parts of the heart, e.g. LV mural thrombus. This is detected in over 40% of cases of acute MI at autopsy. Usually this occurs in the presence of anterior infarction and apical dyskinesis or LV aneurysm. Thrombus can also form in other low-output states, especially with chamber enlargement or where there is foreign material in the heart, e.g. pacing leads, central lines, prosthetic valves, particularly if inadequately anticoagulated or malfunctioning.

2. Examination of the aorta

TTE only gives good images of the ascending aorta, aortic arch and proximal descending aorta in a small minority of adults. TOE can add to this by providing excellent imaging of the aortic root, proximal ascending aorta, distal aortic arch and descending thoracic aorta. The interposition of the trachea between the oesophagus and ascending aorta limits the ability to image the upper ascending aorta and proximal aortic arch.

Aortic dimensions and dilatation

TOE allows accurate determination of aortic dimensions and reveals dilatation seen in aortic aneurysm.

Aortic atheroma

TOE helps detect and differentiate mobile and immobile atheromatous plaques. Mobile plaques may be associated with a higher embolic rate, as are pedunculated rather than linear plaques. Atheromatous plaques in the ascending aorta are found by TOE in at least 1% of individuals who have suffered an embolic CVA.

Aortic dissection (Fig. 5.8)

TOE is the best technique for the diagnosis of aortic dissection, particularly of the ascending aorta where surgical intervention is urgent. TOE makes the diagnosis with sensitivity and specificity around 98%, better than angiography or CT scanning. Dissection of the descending thoracic aorta can also be identified.

3. Endocarditis

TTE should always be used in the initial assessment of suspected or definite endocarditis. The superior spatial resolution provided by TOE allows small

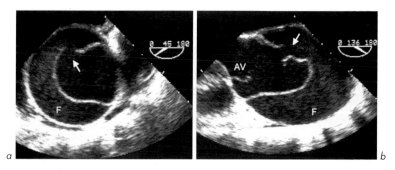

a *b*

Fig. 5.8 *Dissecting aneurysm of the aortic root and ascending aorta – TOE.* **(a)** *Short-axis view and* **(b)** *long-axis view of the ascending aorta showing dissection intimal flap with entry point (arrow). There is spontaneous contrast in the false lumen (F).*

vegetations of only 1–2 mm to be identified and their location and morphology to be examined. All valves can be examined, but TOE is especially useful for the mitral and aortic valves (right-sided vegetations are often large and can be detected by TTE). In aortic subacute bacterial endocarditis (SBE), TOE is especially useful for aortic root abscess (TOE shows over 85% of such cases, TTE less than 30%), fistula or aneurysm of the sinus of Valsalva.

TOE is of use in endocarditis:

- Where TTE has not been diagnostic
- To assess the size, location and morphology of vegetations
- To assess possible complications such as aortic root abscess.

TOE should be considered in the majority of cases of suspected endocarditis.

4. Native valve assessment

Mitral valve

TTE is good but some aspects may be hard to assess. The posterior leaflet may be poorly visualized, especially if calcified or in the presence of mitral annular calcification. TOE can provide essential information in planning intervention such as MV repair (Figs 5.9 and 5.10).

In MR, quantitative assessment of severity by TTE is difficult. TOE allows a more thorough assessment by Doppler and colour flow of the degree of MR

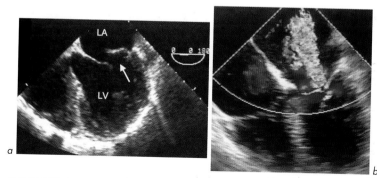

Fig. 5.9 TOE showing **(a)** severe prolapse of posterior mitral valve leaflet (arrow) and **(b)** severe mitral regurgitation.

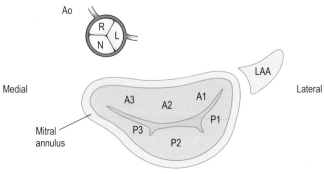

a **Transthoracic**

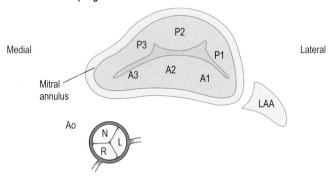

b **Transoesophageal**

Fig. 5.10 *Mitral valve viewed from (a) transthoracic parasternal view and (b) transoesophageal mid-gastric view. The 3 scallops of the anterior (A1, A2, A3) and posterior (P1, P2, P3) leaflets, the left atrial appendage (LAA) and the position of the proximal aorta (Ao) are shown. N = non-coronary sinus, R = right coronary sinus, L = left coronary sinus.*

within the LA. Severity can also be assessed by the pattern of pulmonary venous flow (severe MR may be associated with reversal of flow). The morphology of the valve can be examined to assess if suitable for valve repair rather than replacement. The exact segment of the valve which is causing regurgitation can be identified.

TOE can be used intraoperatively to assess the adequacy of valve repair.

In MS, TOE is very useful in deciding if a stenosed mitral valve is suitable for balloon valvuloplasty or whether surgical treatment such as mitral valvotomy or replacement is needed.

Balloon valvuloplasty for MS is **not** suitable if:

- The anterior MV leaflet is immobile, thickened or calcified
- The chordae are thickened or calcified
- The leaflet tips are heavily calcified
- There is more than mild MR
- There is visible thrombus (e.g. in LA appendage).

Aortic valve

TOE allows confident prediction of the integrity and number of cusps, evaluation of the aortic root, aortic sinuses and LVOT. Morphological assessment of AV can help give an indication of the aetiology of AR and colour flow mapping gives an indication of severity.

Tricuspid and pulmonary valves and right heart

The TV does not lend itself particularly well to TOE. Views can be obtained, but TTE is often sufficient. The PV, right ventricular outflow tract (RVOT) and proximal pulmonary artery can also be imaged reasonably well by TOE. It is often possible to view the 4 pulmonary veins and their connections with the LA, or to determine if there is partial or total anomalous pulmonary venous drainage.

5. Prosthetic valve assessment (see section 6.3)

This is one of the most important indications for TOE. The close proximity of the transducer to the valve, the reduction in interfering tissues nearby and enhanced spatial resolution make this very useful and superior to TTE.

The MV position is particularly well examined because of the orientation relative to the transducer. Paravalvular MR is well detected and may occur in up to 2.5% of all MV prostheses. TOE can be used intraoperatively and postoperatively to assess the presence and severity of paraprosthetic MR. TOE is useful in distinguishing between mild, moderate and severe paraprosthetic MR (the latter may deteriorate progressively and require re-operation). Shadowing of the LVOT occurs with mitral prostheses and may limit the ability to detect AR.

For aortic prostheses, TOE also has advantages over TTE, especially in biological valve degeneration, obstruction of prosthesis, regurgitation, abscesses

141

or mass lesions (vegetations, thrombus). There are still some limitations even with TOE. The imaging planes are limited and as a result the acoustic shadow generated by mechanical prostheses may hide lesions in some areas. Aortic prostheses leave a portion of the aortic annulus immune from interrogation which may lead to underdiagnosis of root abscess.

6. Congenital disease (see section 6.4)

TOE plays an important role, especially in paediatric practice and in complex congenital heart disease. It may help diagnose and assess severity and haemodynamics in:

- Intracardiac shunts – PFO, ASD (Fig. 5.11), VSD
- Extracardiac shunt – PDA
- Congenital valvular abnormalities
- Aortic coarctation
- Anomalous systemic or pulmonary venous connections
- Follow-up of corrective or palliative procedures.

7. Cardiac and paracardiac masses (see section 6.1)

TOE is superior to TTE in a number of settings and should be considered if TTE does not adequately visualize masses, particularly in:

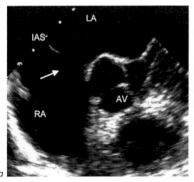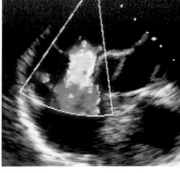

Fig. 5.11 Ostium secundum ASD. **(a)** Defect in interatrial septum (IAS) measuring 16 mm shown at TOE examination (arrow). **(b)** Colour flow mapping showing flow from left to right atrium.

- LA and appendage
- Descending thoracic aorta
- Pericardium
- PA
- Right-sided paracardiac region
- SVC and IVC
- Anterior mediastinum.

5.2 STRESS ECHO

Stress transthoracic echo aids in the diagnosis of ischaemic heart disease. It helps to localize the site and quantifies the extent of ischaemia by the demonstration of regional wall motion and thickness abnormalities with stress which are not present at rest (Figs 5.12 and 5.13). This technique may be used as an alternative to exercise stress ECG testing or stress radionuclide myocardial perfusion scanning (e.g. stress thallium) in certain circumstances. Stress may be either by:

- Physical exercise (treadmill or bicycle)
- Pharmacological means (by the continuous infusion of an agent such as the vasodilating inotropic agent dobutamine or vasodilators which divert blood from areas served by stenosed arteries to other regions, e.g. dipyridamole or adenosine)
- Temporary cardiac pacing (used to increase heart rate, but invasive).

The sensitivity of stress echo is around 80% and the specificity around 90%. These compare favourably with exercise ECG testing which has a sensitivity of around 70% and a specificity of around 80%.

Stress echo is also used in some centres to determine the extent of LVOTO associated with HCM when septal ablation by catheter instillation of ethanol or surgical myomectomy are being considered. A resting LVOT gradient of 30 mmHg in these cases may increase to over 100 mmHg during stress and may indicate the need for septal reduction.

Indications for stress echo

Ischaemic heart disease (Fig. 5.12)

1. Uncertain diagnosis, equivocal exercise stress ECG test
2. Inability to exercise on treadmill

Parasternal long-axis view

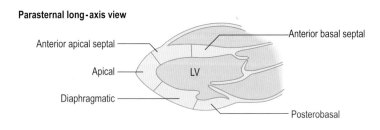

Anterior apical septal

Apical

Diaphragmatic

Anterior basal septal

LV

Posterobasal

Apical 4-chamber view

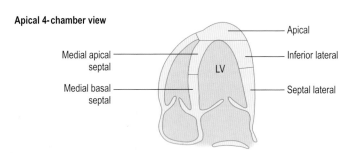

Medial apical
septal

Medial basal
septal

Apical

Inferior lateral

LV

Septal lateral

Parasternal short-axis – MV level

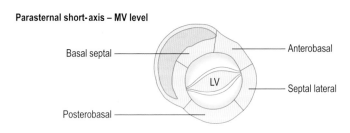

Basal septal

Posterobasal

Anterobasal

LV

Septal lateral

Parasternal short-axis – papillary muscle level

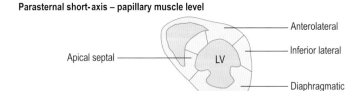

Apical septal

Anterolateral

Inferior lateral

LV

Diaphragmatic

Fig. 5.12 *16-segment model of left ventricular myocardium. This model is appropriate for studies assessing wall motion, as the tip of the apex does not move. Adapted from Schiller et al J Am Soc Echocardiogr 1989; 2:358–367.*

3. Resting ECG abnormality prevents interpretation of changes with exercise (e.g. LBBB, LVH with strain, digoxin)
4. Following acute MI
5. Localization of site of ischaemia
6. Assessment of myocardial viability – hibernation or stunning
7. Evaluation following revascularization (e.g. PCI ± stent or CABG)
8. Stress echo is especially useful in the assessment of possible ischaemic heart disease:
   - In women with chest pain and cardiovascular risk factors
   - Following heart transplantation
   - Prior to renal transplantation
   - Prior to vascular surgery.

LVOTO

1. HCM – to assess the LVOTO gradient with stress when considering septal ablation or resection
2. Upper septal bulge. Seen in elderly subjects due to fibrosis and hypertrophy. Unusually causes LVOTO.

Assessment of changes in cardiac haemodynamics with stress

1. Valve area and pressure difference, e.g. AV area in calcific AS
2. Severity of valvular regurgitation, e.g. MR
3. PASP, e.g. in MS or MR
4. Pressure difference across stenosis in aortic coarctation
5. HCM to assess LVOTO.

Limitations of stress echo

- Failure to achieve adequate workload
- Poor endocardial definition – helped by contrast echo techniques
- Complications of procedure.

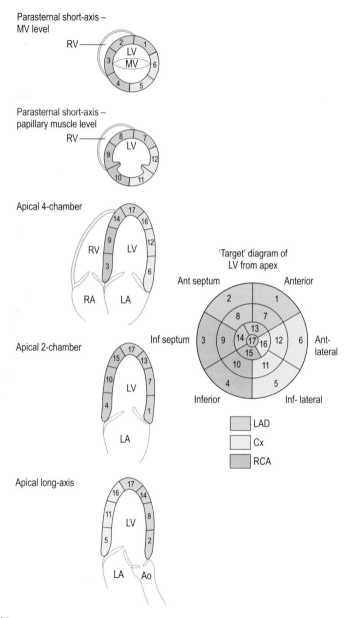

Parasternal short-axis – MV level

RV — LV MV

Parasternal short-axis – papillary muscle level

RV — LV

Apical 4-chamber

RV LV RA LA

Apical 2-chamber

LV LA

Apical long-axis

LV LA Ao

'Target' diagram of LV from apex

Ant septum   Anterior

Inf septum   Ant-lateral

Inferior   Inf-lateral

LAD
Cx
RCA

(left) Fig. 5.13 17-segment model of left ventricular myocardium. Differs from 16-segment model by addition of apical cap (segment 17), imaging of which has improved with contrast and harmonic echo. Used predominantly for myocardial perfusion studies or to compare with other imaging modalities (e.g. cardiac CT or MRI). Arterial territories are shown: LAD = left anterior descending, Cx = circumflex, RCA = right coronary artery. Adapted from Cerueira et al Circulation 2002; 105:539–542.

Complications of stress echo

This is a safe procedure if carried out with care. The rate of major complications is <0.5%.

- Major – sustained VT, sustained SVT, myocardial infarction, hypotension
- Minor – flushing, dizziness, dyspnoea, ectopic beats or non-sustained SVT, anticholinergic side effects with atropine.

5.3 CONTRAST ECHO

Contrast agents can be injected into the bloodstream resulting in increased echogenicity of the blood or myocardium. This can produce opacification of the cardiac chambers or an increase in echogenicity of the myocardium. Ultrasound 'contrast' is generated by the presence of microbubbles. At low ultrasound power outputs, microbubbles scatter ultrasound at the gas–liquid interface, resulting in detection of a reflected signal by the transducer. In addition, ultrasound causes compression and expansion, i.e. oscillation, of microbubbles. The resonant frequency of a microbubble is related to its diameter. Harmonic imaging can detect this nonlinear resonant signal. At high power outputs, ultrasound results in microbubble destruction. Careful adjustment of instrument power output is needed during contrast echo.

Echo contrast agents

There are two types of echo contrast agent:

1. Those that opacify the right heart
2. Those that opacify the left heart and myocardium.

When the size of the microbubbles is greater then the pulmonary capillary diameter, they are trapped in the capillaries and no contrast enters the left side of the heart in the absence of an intracardiac right to left communication. Left heart and myocardial contrast is achieved using microbubbles in the 1–5 μm range, which cross the pulmonary capillary bed. Microbubbles in this size range resonate with frequency 1.5–7 MHz, corresponding to clinical transducer frequencies.

Right heart contrast

The most widely used contrast for right heart studies is agitated saline. A simple approach is rapidly to push 5 mL of sterile saline with a small amount (approximately 0.1 mL) of air or the patient's blood between two syringes connecting with 3-way stop-cock taps. This results in the production of large diameter microbubbles which do not pass through the pulmonary capillary bed. When the saline appears opaque, it is injected rapidly into a peripheral vein during echo imaging. Care must be taken to ensure there is no visible free air in the injection system. Agitated saline should not be used in patients with known significant right to left shunting to avoid the risk of paradoxical embolization into the systemic circulation.

Left heart and myocardial contrast

Left heart and myocardial contrast agents consist of air or low-solubility fluorocarbon gas in stabilized microbubbles encapsulated with agents such as denatured albumin or monosaccharides. These contrasts are usually prepared just before use. Some require re-suspension before intravenous injection while others are diluted and given as a continuous infusion. Microbubbles are fragile, so careful handling and infusion techniques are needed. The optimum volume and infusion rate depend on the specific contrast agent used, to provide full opacification while minimizing attenuation due to excess microbubble density.

Applications of contrast echo

The main clinical applications of echo contrast studies are:
1. Detection of intracardiac shunt
2. LV opacification
3. Myocardial perfusion
4. Enhancement of Doppler signals.

1. Detection of intracardiac shunt. Right heart contrast allows the detection of a right to left intracardiac shunt. With a patent foramen ovale (PFO), shunting may be seen only after a Valsalva manoeuvre because of the transient increase in RA compared to LA pressure (Fig. 6.14). Even with a predominant left to right shunt, e.g. with an atrial septal defect, there is usually a small amount of right to left shunting when the pressures on both sides equalize, allowing detection of the shunt with right heart contrast. Right heart contrast may also be used to identify a left-sided superior vena cava or to demonstrate the systemic venous inflow pathway in complex congenital heart disease.

2. LV opacification in patients with poor image quality on resting studies or during stress echo enhances the identification of wall motion abnormalities and overall LV systolic function. Endocardial border detection can be enhanced (e.g. for examination of LV dyssynchrony for CRT assessment). Most centres now routinely perform contrast enhancement during stress studies when endocardial definition is suboptimal.

3. Myocardial perfusion with contrast echo is technically challenging. Only approximately 6% of LV stroke volume perfuses the myocardium via the coronary arteries, so the relative number of microbubbles in the coronary circulation reaching the myocardium is small. Mechanical and ultrasound destruction of microbubbles further limits contrast echo. This can be used to assess myocardial perfusion, viability and function in acute MI or during bypass surgery and during stress echo. Contrast can be injected directly into a coronary artery in certain situations (Fig. 5.14). Myocardial perfusion by echo contrast has not yet become a routine clinical test.

4. Enhancement of Doppler signals. Contrast may be used to increase Doppler signal strength, e.g. a TR jet to estimate PASP. The effect of contrast on the Doppler signal varies with instruments and this approach has not gained widespread use.

Limitations of contrast echo

- Right heart contrast to detect large intracardiac shunts is infrequently needed, given the sensitivity of colour Doppler and TOE. The primary use of right heart contrast is for detection of a PFO. A small ventricular septal defect usually will not be detected with right heart contrast injection because there is little right to left shunting.
- The use of left heart contrast requires considerable experience to judge the infusion rate and volume needed to opacify the LV optimally. When the

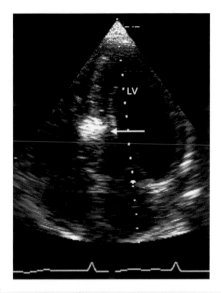

Fig. 5.14 *Contrast echo study in a subject with hypertrophic cardiomyopathy. Contrast has been selectively injected into the 1st septal branch of the left anterior descending coronary artery during cardiac catheterization and can be seen in the septum (arrow) on apical 4-chamber echo. This shows the area of myocardium that is infarcted by the technique of selective instillation of ethanol ('septal reduction').*

microbubble density is too high an excessive contrast effect at the apex results in attenuation of signal or shadowing of the rest of the LV. A swirling appearance may be seen with too little contrast or in low flow states. Bubble destruction may result in a swirling pattern with inadequate ventricular opacification.

- The addition of contrast injection to the echo examination increases the cost, duration and risk of the procedure.
- Contrast during a standard echo or stress echo study may make this approach impractical in many laboratories due to the time and personnel needed.
- Adverse reactions to contrast agents may occur, such as nausea, vomiting, headaches, flushing and dizziness. Major reactions such as hypersensitivity or anaphylaxis are rare.

5.4 THREE-DIMENSIONAL (3-D) ECHO

Advances in echo technology now allow the generation of 3-D echo images. This refers to several approaches for the acquisition and display of ultrasound images. 3-D echo allows the heart to be seen in new ways showing complex and anatomical features not possible with standard 2-D echo. Cardiac structures can be rotated or viewed from different orientations even after image acquisition. This ability to view anatomy from different viewpoints is an advantage.

3-D ultrasound is not a new concept and has been known as a clinical application in noncardiac applications such as obstetrics for over 10 years. To be clinically useful, cardiac imaging requires high time resolution to keep up with heart movement. Previously 3-D echo involved reconstruction from multiple 2-D images. New triggering technology and high frame rate processing have allowed the development of live (real-time) 3-D echo. It is likely that much of echo will become fully 3-D in the future, but the optimum 3-D approach is evolving.

Real-time (live) 3-D echo techniques are now available which allow transthoracic and transoesophageal echo (TOE or TEE) studies. In some centres these are used before and during cardiac surgery.

With improved technical issues, live 3-D echo can impact upon patient care and improve pre-surgical planning. It is also a valuable method of communicating information to surgeons, physicians and patients. 3-D echo is particularly helpful for evaluation of valvular abnormalities such as before and during MV repair or percutaneous mitral balloon valvuloplasty and congenital heart disease. Although 3-D echo is not yet in widespread clinical use, it has a number of clinical applications, including:

- Enhanced diagnostic capability reducing or eliminating the need for expensive or invasive tests and procedures
- Better visualization of the heart to improve surgical planning and provide intraoperative information
- Information about cardiac haemodynamics (e.g. LV function)
- Live assessments of heart valve function
- Examination of complex congenital heart abnormalities
- Teaching and research.

The basic approaches to displaying 3-D echo data are:
- Real-time 3-D display
- Simultaneous 2-D image planes
- Border reconstructions.

The most intuitive is a 3-D image that can be rotated and viewed from multiple angles in real-time. Current display formats suffer from showing 3-D images on 2-D displays. This limitation should be resolved as 3-D display systems become more widely available. 3-D echo can also be used to generate multiple 2-D image planes. As with 2-D echo, quantification from 3-D echo requires the tracing of cardiac borders. This can provide very accurate LV volume measurements and can allow detailed assessments of wall motion, myocardial thickening and LV shape. Border tracing is time-consuming and as automated edge detection programs improve, analysis time will decrease and this will become more widely used clinically.

Clinical applications of 3-D echo

1. Chamber quantification

- Quantification of ventricular volumes and function. Measurements of volume throughout the cardiac cycle, LV mass and dimensions of LV and RV. Analysis of global and regional wall motion. 3-D echo is superior to 2-D echo for both LV and RV volumes. The technique requires acquisition of 3-D echo data and manual endocardial border tracing. Since the process of tracing is time-consuming, semi-automated techniques and detection algorithms are being developed. The advent of real-time volumetric scanning will enhance the use of 3-D echo in volume measurement.
- Infarct size estimation.
- Evaluation of distorted ventricles.
- Serial LV volume measurements in individuals with valvular regurgitation to help time surgery (e.g. AR, MR).
- Assessment of RV function. This is limited by 2-D echo because of anatomical considerations including the asymmetrical pyramidal shape of RV which does not conform to simple geometrical assumptions.
- Assessment of ventricular function in congenital cardiac lesions such as ASD and VSD.
- May be useful in assessment of patients with heart failure for CRT.
- LA volume measurement.

2. Valvular heart disease

- Real-time 3-D echo obviates many of the practical limitations in reconstructive 3-D techniques and also provides greater clinical applications in valvular heart disease, both in diagnostic evaluation and in real-time guidance during surgical valve repair.

- 3-D echo is ideally suited for assessing valve function given the non-planar anatomy of the cardiac valves and the complex anatomical changes seen in valvular heart disease.

- MV is particularly suited because of the complex relationship between the valve leaflets, subvalvular apparatus and myocardial wall. 3-D echo can give insights into MV structure and assessment of MV prolapse, endocarditis and congenital MV abnormalities. Important functional and anatomical information can be gained in ischaemic and functional MR resulting from derangement of the normal relationship between MV leaflets, annulus and LV. The technique is useful in guiding surgical repair of the MV. Real-time 3-D images can be rotated and cropped at different levels to show different views. For example, MV can be viewed from the perspective of the LA. This is helpful for surgeons during MV repair. Real-time 3-D is useful in quantifying MR and reconstruction of jets. It can be used for assessment of MS (Fig. 5.15) and calculation of MV area. 3-D echo has been used for guidance of percutaneous mitral valvuloplasty.

- AV. 3-D echo has been applied for anatomical assessment of AV and root morphology and to calculate valve area. It shows aortic flow patterns and quantifies AR. AV vegetations can be localized. Congenital outflow obstruction can be demonstrated, as can outflow changes in AV after balloon dilatation. AV can be viewed from the perspective of the aorta.

- TV and PV. 3-D echo has been used to show abnormalities in rheumatic and degenerative TV and PV disease and allows reconstruction of congenital TV abnormalities such as AV canal defects and assessment of PV stenosis.

- Determination of the size of vegetations in endocarditis.

3. Congenital heart disease

- ASD. The size, shape and location of defects and their relationship to surrounding tissues and the extent of residual surrounding tissue can be assessed. In secundum ASDs the extent of the retro-aortic rim often determines the feasibility of percutaneous device closure and 3-D echo can demonstrate successful closure.

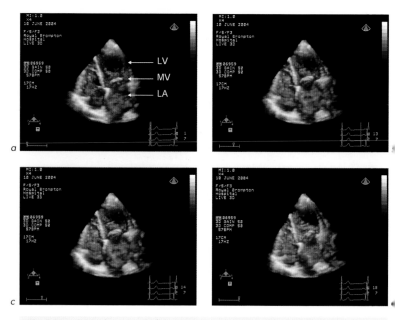

Fig 5.15 *3-D echo. Images from a study in a patient with mitral stenosis.*

- VSD. Visualization of the entire septum is an advantage to assess the size and shape of the defect and jet using colour flow techniques.
- LV and RV size and function can be assessed in patients with congenital heart disease.
- Circumferential extent of subaortic membranes can be visualized.
- Congenital valvular malformations (e.g. MV) can be examined.

4. Intraoperative

- MV prolapse repair, to assess anatomy, guide surgical repair and final adequacy of repair.
- Surgery for congenital heart lesions.
- HOCM during septal myomectomy to show the extent of septal thickening, LVOTO, MV systolic anterior motion and post-procedure result.
- Guide catheters into the 3-D space without X-ray exposure, e.g. during EPS.

5. Aortic disease

- Define the anatomy of aortic dissection.

6. Contrast echo

- Improve quantification of LV volume and function.
- Evaluation of myocardial perfusion. Ability to record the entire LV and quantify the full extent of hypoperfused myocardium. The problem of microbubble destruction, even with triggered imaging, remains a challenge.

7. Tagging and tracking the LV surface in real-time

This helps in the quantification of myocardial mechanics and shows changes in regional shape and strain. The approach has potential and may have comparable uses and similar quantitative ability to cardiac MRI. The superior temporal resolution of echo should offer unique advantages. In the future, combining the greater temporal resolution of 3-D echo with the excellent spatial resolution of MRI or CT may yield excellent imaging techniques ('fusion imaging') providing anatomical and physiological information.

8. Teaching of cardiac anatomy and physiology and research

Limitations of 3-D echo

Despite the potential for 3-D echo, the technique is not yet in widespread clinical use. This is due to several factors:

- 3-D echo may only visualize what can also be seen on a good 2-D echo study. Thus, an expert echocardiographer can obtain similar information from a conventional examination without the need for costly instrumentation and long post-processing times.
- Operator instruction and experience in 3-D echo is necessary.
- 3-D echo image quality depends on the quality of 2-D images for the ability to obtain motion and artefact free 3-D data.
- 3-D echo can only create a virtual sense of depth on a flat 2-D screen.
- Some 3-D echo techniques such as manual endocardial contour tracing are time-consuming.
- Some of the technology remains expensive.

Some of these limitations will be overcome with newer techniques. With rapid advances in digital image processing, 3-D echo is probably at the beginning of its evolution. The incorporation of 3-D technology into conventional echo systems with operator-friendly applications is reducing the time and effort required to obtain 3-D images. Standard 3-D echo protocols are being developed. Further advances in real-time 3-D echo with real-time colour echo, contrast echo, tissue Doppler imaging and intracardiac ultrasound may be beneficial.

Ongoing and future developments in 3-D echo

These include:

1. Technological advances and expanding clinical applications
2. Automated surface detection and quantification
3. Single heartbeat full volume acquisition
4. Improvements in transthoracic and TOE real-time 3-D imaging.

These and other echo techniques will undoubtedly find clinical use, but the existing echo techniques described in this book are very powerful and will continue to have important clinical uses.

5.5 ECHO IN SPECIAL HOSPITAL SETTINGS

Echo can be of great benefit in a number of special hospital situations:

- Preoperative
- Intraoperative
- Intensive care unit (ICU), coronary care unit (CCU), cardiac catheter laboratory
- Accident & Emergency (A&E) department
- Portable (hand-held) echo.

Preoperative echo

Echo can help in the preoperative assessment of patients undergoing cardiac and noncardiac surgery. There are internationally published guidelines including those by the American College of Cardiology, American Heart Association and European Society of Cardiology relating to echo assessment for preoperative patients. For noncardiac surgery, particularly in high-risk operations such as orthopaedic or vascular surgery, echo can be used to assess LV systolic function or valvular function. Myocardial perfusion can be assessed by stress echo. Preoperative echo should be used for cardiac surgery and for orthopaedic, vascular, major and genitourinary surgery.

156

Cardiac risk for noncardiac surgical procedures (death, MI)

High >5%

- Emergency major surgery, particularly in older individuals
- Aortic and other major vascular surgery
- Peripheral vascular surgery
- Anticipated prolonged surgery with significant blood loss and/or fluid shifts

Medium <5%

- Carotid endarterectomy
- Head and neck surgery
- Intraperitoneal surgery
- Intrathoracic surgery
- Orthopaedic surgery
- Urological surgery

Low <1%

- Endoscopic procedures
- Superficial procedures
- Cataract surgery
- Breast surgery

Adapted from Eagle et al *Circulation* 2002; 105:1257–1267.

Specific uses of preoperative echo in cardiac and noncardiac high-risk surgery

- Assessment of LV function – global, regional wall motion abnormalities, stress echo for demonstration of myocardial ischaemia
- MV assessment – need for valve operation and severity of MR or MS, suitability for MV repair, suitability for balloon valvuloplasty, mitral annular calcification
- AV assessment – AS and severity, suitability of AV replacement and prediction of annular size and LVOT size
- Pulmonary hypertension and right heart assessment
- Aortic atheroma
- Thoracic aortic aneurysm.

Clinical predictors of increased perioperative cardiovascular risk (death, MI, HF)

High
- Unstable coronary syndromes – recent (under 30 days) or acute (under 7 days) MI, unstable or severe angina (Canadian class III or IV)
- Decompensated heart failure
- Significant arrhythmia – high-level AV block, symptomatic ventricular arrhythmia with underlying heart disease, SVTs with poorly-controlled ventricular rate
- Severe valvular abnormality

Medium
- Mild angina (Canadian class I or II)
- Previous MI
- Compensated or previous heart failure
- Diabetes mellitus
- Renal insufficiency

Low
- Advanced age
- Abnormal ECG – LVH, LBBB, ST-T abnormalities
- Low functional capacity
- Previous stroke
- Uncontrolled hypertension

Adapted from Eagle et al *Circulation* 2002; 105:1257–1267.

Intraoperative echo

The use of intraoperative echo has increased in adult and paediatric surgery. This refers mainly to intraoperative TOE particularly for cardiac surgery, but this is also used in some high-risk noncardiac operations. This technique can help in the acquisition of new information (12–38% of cases) during operation and may impact upon treatment (9–14% of cases).

Intraoperative TOE is not without risk and is an independent predictor of postoperative dysphagia (over 7-times greater odds in a study of 838 patients, but another study of 7200 patients showed no increased mortality and only 0.2% morbidity).

Uses of intraoperative TOE (from Cheitlin et al 2003, ACC/AHA Practice Guidelines)

- MV repair. Detailed anatomical evaluation and adequacy of repair (residual MR, systolic anterior motion and dynamic LVOTO, iatrogenic MS)
- MV replacement – valve sizing, adequacy or replacement, paravalvular MR (jets are more common after MV than AV replacements), chordal interference with valvular function
- Ventricular function – LV (regional, global) and RV
- AV replacement – valve sizing, adequacy of replacement, prosthesis size mismatch, paravalvular AR, LVOTO
- Congenital heart lesion repairs (e.g. transposition of the great arteries) – detection of residual defects after surgery, such as residual shunt, in 4.4–12.8% of cases, baffle interrogation, RV function
- Intracardiac air – intracavity, myocardial, adequacy of de-airing after bypass
- Surgical myomectomy for HOCM – residual LVOTO, acquired VSD, coronary fistula
- Aortic atheroma
- Minimally invasive cardiac surgery
- Coronary artery bypass surgery.

Coronary care unit/intensive care unit/A&E/cardiac catheter laboratory

There is a role for transthoracic echo and TOE. Examples include:
- Size of pericardial effusion, echo features of tamponade
- Pericardiocentesis – echo-guided assistance with placement of drainage catheter
- LV regional wall motion abnormalities in acute myocardial infarction
- Valvular abnormalities
- Assessment of endocarditis or pyrexia of unknown origin (e.g. TOE to exclude endocarditis in an ICU patient with unexplained fever and *Staphylococcus aureus* in blood cultures)
- Assessment of the patient following major trauma
- Mitral balloon valvuloplasty
- Catheter placement during electrophysiological studies and arrhythmia ablation.

Portable or hand-held echo

This refers to the use of small, lightweight, portable echo machines, which can be used in different locations at the patient's bedside (Fig. 5.16). These vary in their levels of complexity from very simple pocket-size instruments to larger instruments the size of a laptop computer or briefcase with many features of larger machines. Some have limited capability with a single transducer producing 2-D images and others have more modalities including 2-D, M-mode, pulsed wave and continuous wave Doppler and colour flow imaging. Some support multiple echo transducers and have sophisticated functions such as TOE. These instruments can be used in situations such as the A&E department, coronary care unit and cardiology outpatients clinic. Some devices will operate from a battery source and can be used outside the hospital, for example at the scene of a trauma incident. There needs to be careful local evaluation of the clinical indications and quality assurance in the use of these devices in each medical centre, to monitor diagnostic accuracy.

Clinical uses of portable echo

- Rapid assessment of patients in the A&E department, ICU, CCU and cardiac catheter laboratory

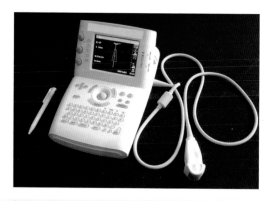

Fig. 5.16 Portable echocardiogram machine. The mass is under 3 kg. Pen shown for scale is 14 cm long.

- Exclusion of pericardial effusion and/or echo features of tamponade in trauma patients
- Assessment of LV and RV systolic function
- Regional wall motion abnormalities
- Identification of valvular abnormalities such as AS or MR
- Assessment of patients with hypertension to determine if there is LVH
- Assessment of patients with chest pain and non-diagnostic ECG where an akinetic LV segment may indicate acute myocardial infarction, whereas a pericardial effusion may indicate pericarditis
- Assessment of patients with hypotension, where a small hyperdynamic LV may suggest septicaemic shock while a dilated poor LV may suggest a primary cardiac abnormality
- Portable echo can in some situations be a useful supplement to the physical examination.

Limitations of portable echo

- Appropriate training and experience is needed for any echo assessment
- Misdiagnosis due to the limitation of instruments giving suboptimal image quality and inexperienced operator
- If an abnormality is suggested then a full echo examination may be needed with standard equipment.

Intracardiac echo

This uses a catheter-like ultrasound probe which is passed to the right heart from the femoral vein. The frequency used is 5–10 MHz. This allows ultrasound penetration of tissues up to 10 cm from the transducer. At present, devices provide single-plane imaging with pulsed wave and colour Doppler using a steerable transducer connected to standard echo equipment.

The tip of the transducer can be placed in the inferior vena cava, RA and RV. The RA is often the most useful location for monitoring invasive procedures. From the RA, it is possible to obtain echo views of the AV, MV, TV, LV and RV, as well as the interatrial septum, LA and pulmonary veins. From the inferior vena cava the transducer can be used to visualize the abdominal aorta.

Clinical uses of intracardiac echo

This is used primarily for monitoring invasive procedures in the cardiac catheter laboratory, although the clinical utility of this technique has not been fully evaluated. Intracardiac echo may be used because the image quality with transthoracic echo is usually suboptimal in these situations. It may be used as an alternative to TOE during invasive procedures, as TOE often requires general anaesthesia because of the duration of the procedure. Intracardiac echo is well tolerated and provides accurate continuous information to the physician carrying out the procedure.

The primary applications of intracardiac echo are in monitoring during:
- Percutaneous device closure of defects – e.g. ASD
- Balloon valvuloplasty – e.g. MS
- Electrophysiological studies (EPS) – e.g. catheter ablation procedures for arrhythmias.

For device closures, this technique can be used to evaluate the defect at baseline and identify adjacent structures such as pulmonary veins. During the procedure, the technique can be used to help position the closure device optimally. After the procedure, Doppler and colour flow mapping can be used to examine for any residual shunt.

In EPS, intracardiac echo can be used to:
- Monitor trans-septal puncture
- Give detailed evaluation of LA and pulmonary vein anatomy
- Allow placement of the ablation probe with optimum tissue contact
- Monitor the development of spontaneous echo contrast during ablation
- Detect complications such as intracardiac thrombus, pericardial effusion or pulmonary vein obstruction.

Limitations of intracardiac echo

- Cost. Disposable catheters are expensive.
- Risks of invasive procedure. However, most patients are already having an invasive procedure and there is a little additional risk.
- Image quality. Biplane or multiplane probe will improve image acquisition.

Intravascular ultrasound (IVUS)

This is performed using an intravascular steerable catheter that is positioned within the coronary arteries during interventional coronary procedures. The ultrasound frequency used is 30–50 MHz. The transducer provides an image depth of 2–3 cm with high resolution into the vessel wall and atherosclerotic plaques. A small dedicated ultrasound system is usually used to acquire the images. The catheter is positioned by the interventional cardiologist during the procedure.

Intravascular ultrasound may be useful when standard angiographic data do not give full information regarding the length or severity of a coronary artery narrowing and the condition of the atherosclerotic plaque. This information can then be used to plan further treatment.

CHAPTER 6

Cardiac masses, infection, congenital abnormalities

6.1 CARDIAC MASSES

Echo is very important in detecting cardiac masses and giving an indication of their nature. Masses include:

- Tumours (primary or secondary)
- Blood clot (thrombus)
- Infected material (vegetation or abscess)
- Artificial (prosthetic) valves and pacing wires.

1. Tumours of the heart

Echo can detect the site, size, mobility, number and attachment of tumours. This is especially helpful when planning surgical treatment.

Secondary tumours – the majority

These are all malignant since they have metastasized or invaded locally. They are more common than generally realized, occurring in about 10% of all fatal malignancies. The most common primary site is lung (30% of cases of cardiac secondaries – the close proximity plays a role with direct extension to involve the pericardium and heart). Other common primary tumours metastasizing to the heart include breast, kidney, liver, melanoma (this is disproportionately numerous in relation to its total incidence), lymphoma and leukaemia.

Primary tumours – rare

Benign – e.g. myxoma, lipoma, fibroma, rhabdomyoma, papillary fibroelastoma, angioma, paraganglioma, pericardial tumours (pericardial cysts and teratomas).

Malignant – mainly sarcomas – e.g. angiosarcoma (commonest), rhabdomyosarcoma, fibrosarcoma and liposarcoma.

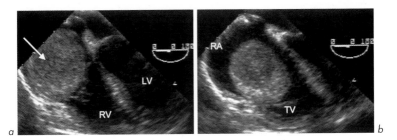

Fig. 6.1 **(a)** *Leiomyosarcoma (arrow) of the inferior vena cava extending into the right atrium.* **(b)** *The mass prolapses through the tricuspid valve. TOE 4-chamber view.*

Echo cannot differentiate between benign and malignant tumours. **2-D echo** shows tumours as echogenic masses within the cavity of the heart, attached to the wall or in the pericardium. The size and mobility can be determined. As with all echo studies, multiple views should be obtained. Occasionally on **M-mode**, a tumour such as myxoma may be seen interfering with valve function (section 2.1). The effects of tumours (e.g. obstruction of valve flow, LV dysfunction due to infiltration or obstruction or pericardial effusion) can also be seen on echo (Fig. 6.1).

Myxoma

Myxomas are rare and occur in the atria or ventricles. They are gelatinous and friable (bits can break away and embolize).
- Single or rarely multiple
- Any age or sex but commonest in middle-aged women
- Most commonly in LA (3 times more common than RA) attached to foramen ovale margin (>80%) and rarely in RV or LV
- The myxoma has a base which is either thin like a stalk or broad
- Myxomas are always attached to either the interatrial or interventricular septum.

Although benign in the neoplastic sense, they are far from benign in their effects. They are slow growing over years and, if untreated, usually fatal.

The effects of myxomas relate to:

- Local cardiac effects (e.g. obstruction of MV which can be sudden and fatal)
- Thromboembolic effects
- Neoplastic effects – fever (pyrexia of unknown origin), weight loss, anaemia, arthralgia, Raynaud's phenomenon, high erythrocyte sedimentation rate (ESR).

Myxomas usually present in one of four ways, in decreasing order of frequency:

1. Breathlessness
2. Systemic emboli
3. Constitutional upset
4. Sudden death (occlusion of MV orifice).

Myxomas may be readily detected by **M-mode** or **2-D echo** (Fig. 6.2). The myxoma can be seen as a mass in the LA cavity and may prolapse through the MV into the LV cavity during diastole obstructing flow. It may be so large as to fill the LA. **Doppler** can show the haemodynamic effects.

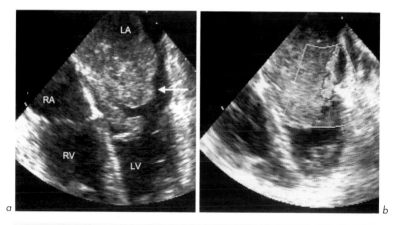

Fig. 6.2 (a) Left atrial myxoma (arrow) shown on TOE 4-chamber view. The tumour is large and lobulated with a broad base attaching it to the interatrial septum. It can be seen to prolapse through the mitral valve. **(b)** It is producing a marked space-occupying effect and causing restriction of flow within the left atrium.

Myxomas very rarely occur in an autosomal dominant familial fashion associated with lentiginosis (multiple freckles) or HCM and so it is wise to screen all first-degree relatives by echo (section 7.6).

Pericardial cysts

These are the most common primary pericardial tumours and are often detected in middle age as an incidental finding during chest X-ray or echo performed for another indication. They can occur anywhere in the pericardium and are masses with echo-free centres attached to the pericardium and with intact walls separating them from the LV cavity. They are benign.

2. Thrombus

This may occur in the ventricular or atrial cavities or walls (mural thrombus). Situations where thrombus formation is increased:

- Dilatation of cardiac chambers
- Reduced wall contractility
- Obstruction and stagnation of flow.

Some examples of these situations include:

- Dilated cardiomyopathy
- Following MI
- LV aneurysm
- LA in valve disease – e.g. MS
- Prosthetic valves
- Arrhythmia – e.g. AF.

2-D imaging is the best echo technique to identify thrombus, which is usually echo-bright. However, this is not always the case and it can be difficult to distinguish from myocardium if they have similar echogenicity. TOE can be helpful, especially for LA and LA appendage thrombus.

False-positive identification of thrombus may occur due to:

- Localized increase in wall thickness
- Tumours
- Dense echoes due to stagnation of blood in an enlarged chamber.

The following favour the diagnosis of thrombus:

167

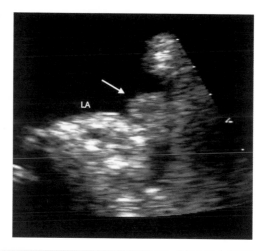

Fig. 6.3 *Left atrial appendage thrombus (arrow).*

1. Mural thrombus may be distinguished from myocardium since myocardium thickens during systole and thrombus does not.
2. Wall motion near a thrombus is nearly always abnormal whereas it is often normal near other pathology, e.g. a tumour.
3. Thrombus usually has a clear identifiable edge which distinguishes it from wall artefact or hazy stagnant blood.
4. Colour flow mapping can distinguish thrombus from stagnant flow.

A number of echo views should always be taken. On 2-D echo, thrombus may be seen as a ball-like or a frond-like mass, or as a well-organized, laminated, raised thickening in the LA or LV. In the LA, there may be associated evidence of sluggish blood flow such as 'spontaneous contrast'. The LA appendage may contain thrombus which can be identified on TOE (Fig. 6.3).

6.2 INFECTION

Endocarditis

This refers to inflammation of any part of the inner layer of the heart, the endocardium, including the heart valves. Inflammatory and/or infected material may accumulate on valves to cause masses called 'vegetations'. These are made up of a mixture of infective material, thrombus, fibrin and red and white blood cells. Vegetations are usually attached on valves but may be on other locations, e.g. chordae, LA, LVOT (HCM), right side of VSD (jet lesion).

The size of vegetations varies from <1 mm to several cm. TTE can miss vegetations <2 mm. TOE may show these, and improves sensitivity to >85%. Large vegetations are particularly associated with fungal infection or endocarditis of the tricuspid valve. Vegetations may be detected by M-mode (section 2.1) or 2-D techniques where they are seen as mobile echo-reflective masses.

There are a number of potential causes which may be infective or non-infective.

Infective

- Bacterial – *Streptococcus*, *Staphylococcus*, Gram-negative bacteria etc.
- Fungal – *Aspergillus*, *Candida*
- Other – *Chlamydia*, *Coxiella*.

Non-infective

- Associated with malignancy (marantic)
- Connective tissue disease – SLE (Libman–Sacks), rheumatoid arthritis
- Acute rheumatic fever (with associated myocarditis and pericarditis).

It is not possible to distinguish by echo alone between infective and non-infective vegetations.

Infective endocarditis

Infection may occur on normal native valves, on previously diseased valves (e.g. rheumatic valves or calcified, degenerative valves) or on artificial (prosthetic) valves.

Endocarditis is a serious condition and potentially life-threatening. It can be acute (e.g. with *Staphylococcus aureus*) or subacute bacterial (SBE). Infection usually follows an episode of bacteraemia, which may not be readily identifiable, or may follow dental treatment or surgery. For this reason it is safest to advise antibiotic prophylaxis treatment for all dental treatment and all surgical procedures for individuals with a known cardiac murmur, congenital lesion, heart valve abnormality or artificial valve. Certain infecting organisms are associated with underlying disease conditions, e.g. *Streptococcus bovis* endocarditis with carcinoma of the colon.

Remember that endocarditis is a *clinical* diagnosis made on the basis of clinical history and examination, blood tests suggesting inflammation and immune complex phenomena and, if possible, culture of the organism from blood. The absence of vegetations on an echo does *not* exclude the diagnosis of endocarditis suspected on clinical grounds. Endocarditis may be present even in the absence of a murmur or fever, especially if antibiotics have been given.

Clinical features supporting endocarditis

- Infection – fever, malaise, night sweats, rigors, anaemia, splenomegaly, clubbing
- Immune complex deposition – microscopic haematuria, vasculitic skin and retinal lesions
- Emboli – in distant organs (brain, retinal, coronary, splenic, renal, femoropopliteal, mesenteric) which may lead to abscess formation
- Cardiac complications:
  1. New or changing murmur(s)
  2. Valve destruction causing regurgitation
  3. Abscess formation around valve rings or in septum causing heart block
  4. Aortic root abscesses which may produce sinus of Valsalva aneurysm or involve coronary ostia
  5. Large vegetations which may obstruct valves (e.g. aortic fungal endocarditis)
  6. Heart failure which may be fatal – due to involvement of the myocardium, pericardial effusion, pyopericardium (pus in the pericardial space, a very serious situation), or valve dysfunction.

Important investigations in endocarditis

- Blood cultures – at least 3 sets from 3 different sites at different times. Up to 90% will be culture positive
- Blood count – raised neutrophil count, normochromic normocytic anaemia
- ESR and C-reactive protein – raised markers of inflammation. Fall accompanies response to treatment
- Immune complex titres raised
- Low complement concentrations
- Urine microscopy – microscopic haematuria

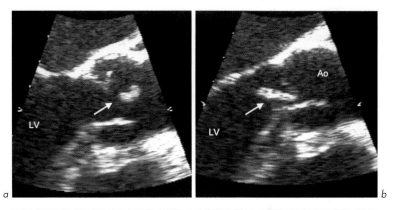

Fig. 6.4 *Endocarditis of the aortic valve showing a large vegetation (arrow).*

- ECG – lengthening of the PR interval suggests aortic root and septal abscess
- Echo – TTE and/or TOE (Fig. 6.4).

Cardiac lesions predisposing to endocarditis

1. Common

- Native valve disease – AV (bicuspid, rheumatic, calcific), MV (regurgitation more often than stenosis, MV prolapse)
- Prosthetic valves
- TV in i.v. drug abusers or after i.v. cannulation (especially large veins)
- Congenital – aortic coarctation, PDA, VSD.

2. Uncommon

- Previously normal valves
- HCM and subaortic stenosis
- Mural thrombus
- Jet lesion
- AV fistula.

3. Rare (virtually never)

- ASD
- Pulmonary stenosis
- Divided PDA.

Antibiotic prophylaxis to prevent endocarditis

The recommended antibiotic regimen should be checked locally and must include attention to a subject's known antibiotic allergies. Used in:

- Known cardiac valve lesion
- Congenital cardiac abnormality – septal defect, PDA
- Prosthetic valve
- Previous endocarditis
- Prevention of recurrence of rheumatic fever

For:

1. Dental treatment
2. Genito-urinary procedures
3. Upper respiratory tract procedures
4. Obstetric, gynaecological and gastrointestinal procedures.

Uses of echo in endocarditis

- Aid diagnosis
- Detect predisposing lesions
- Search for complications
- Response to treatment
- Timing surgical intervention if necessary.

Remember that many vegetations are not seen on TTE until they are >2 mm in size. Colour Doppler may identify AR or MR, acquired VSD or a septal abscess. TOE is very useful in endocarditis, particularly for:

- Visualizing small vegetations
- MV
- Prosthetic valve endocarditis
- Leaflet perforation
- Aortic root abscess
- Sinus of Valsalva aneurysm
- LVOT aneurysm
- LVOT to RA fistula.

Evaluating response to treatment – role for serial echo?

How often serial echos should be done is not clear-cut. Some centres perform weekly echos while antibiotics are being given. It is difficult to justify this routinely unless it will alter clinical management.

Echo can be carried out if there is a deterioration in clinical state of the patient. Vegetations which become smaller may indicate response to treatment – or this may indicate reduced mobility or embolization of part or all of the vegetation! Vegetations getting bigger or new complications (e.g. abscess formation) indicate persistent infection or ineffective treatment.

Timing surgery

Treatment of endocarditis is with antibiotics, usually given for an empirically determined time period of 6 weeks. If an organism is identified, antibiotic therapy can be tailored with known sensitivities. Surgery may be necessary for complications, such as valvular regurgitation or abscess formation. Embolization of infected material may cause cerebral abscesses which need special treatment (antibiotics and surgical drainage).

Echo may detect some indications for surgery in endocarditis

This is not a clear-cut decision and should be based on clinical grounds:

- AR or MR not responding to treatment
- Sinus of Valsalva aneurysm
- Aortic root and septal abscess
- Valve obstruction due to large vegetations
- Failure of antibiotics to control infection or relapse of infection despite changes in antibiotics
- Fungal endocarditis (usually responds best to valve replacement and antifungal treatment)
- Large vegetations with embolic phenomena
- Prosthetic valve endocarditis (usually required).

Consequences and complications of infection

- Spread of vegetations onto other valves or structures, e.g. chordae
- Valvular regurgitation – rupture, prolapse or perforation of valve leaflets or abscess causing regurgitation
- Abscess formation – echo-free space in the perivalvular area (esp. AV) which may cause sinus of Valsalva rupture and left-to-right shunting (often aortic to RA). Abscess in the IVS may cause heart block (usually aortic endocarditis).

Prosthetic valve endocarditis

This can occur on tissue or mechanical valves. Echo can be difficult because of the artefact (reverberation and masking) caused by the prosthesis. It may show vegetations, the complications of infection (e.g. regurgitation) or abscess. TOE may be helpful in making the diagnosis. Endocarditis affecting prosthetic valves is very serious and further valve surgery is often required. It is discussed in the next section.

6.3 ARTIFICIAL (PROSTHETIC) VALVES

These have been used to replace diseased native valves since the 1960s. Although such surgery is still common, attempts are now often made by surgeons to repair valves (particularly the MV) rather than replace them, where possible.

Valves can be positioned to replace any of the 4 native valves. Some patients have more than one prosthetic valve. They may be made of:

- Biological tissue from human or animal valves
- Non-valve tissue material (e.g. pericardium)
- Inert non-biological materials (plastic, metal, carbon, fabric).

A combination of biological tissue and inert material is sometimes used (Fig. 6.5).

1. **Mechanical valves** – Anticoagulation with an agent such as warfarin is necessary to prevent thrombosis:
   - Ball and cage – e.g. Starr–Edwards
   - Tilting disc – one cusp (e.g. Björk–Shiley) or two cusps (e.g. St Jude).
2. **Tissue (biological) valves**
   - Heterograft – from animals
     Porcine – from pigs. Less thrombogenic but less durable than mechanical valves (stenosis or regurgitation usually in 10–15 years). Often have 3 cusps, made of biological tissue fixed by 3 metal stents to a metal sewing ring, e.g. Carpentier–Edwards.
     Bovine – from cattle. Not commonly used; e.g. Ionescu–Shiley valve (bovine pericardial leaflets and titanium frame)
   - Homograft – from humans
     Initially, their lifetime was limited (3 years) but better preservation techniques (e.g. cryopreservation) have increased their usefulness.

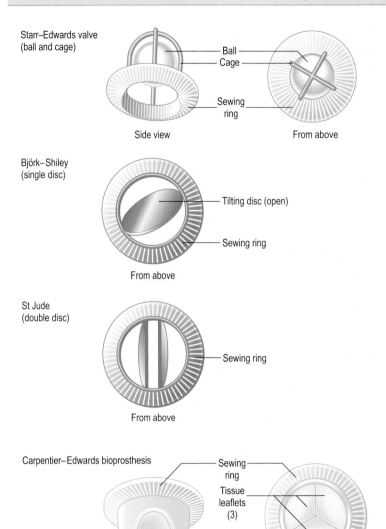

Fig. 6.5 Prosthetic heart valves.

Echo examination of prosthetic valves

Echo can assess:

1. Anatomy – calcification, degeneration, seated correctly or rocking
2. Function:
   - Obstruction – all have some degree of stenosis but this can increase in malfunctioning valves
   - Regurgitation – through valve orifice or paravalvular (due to infection or rocking due to loosening of stitching or degeneration)
3. Infection – valvular, paravalvular abscess
4. Thrombosis.

Examination can be difficult because prosthetic valves:
- Have varied and specialized structures
- Are usually highly echogenic (especially mechanical valves). They may produce echo artefacts such as very bright echo reflection (termed reverberation). They also cast an acoustic shadow that masks or obscures deeper structures.

Following valve replacement surgery, a baseline echo study is often performed after a few weeks. Serial examinations may be performed at intervals after surgery (section 7.6). The type and size of valve should be on the echo request form. As indicated earlier, TOE is an important supplement to TTE in examining prosthetic valves.

M-mode can give some characteristic appearances:

- A Starr–Edwards valve typically shows 2 dense, almost parallel, echo lines representing the sewing ring and the cage. Only echo reflections from the anterior surface of the ball are seen and are traced as dense lines. In the open position, the reflection from the ball moves as far as the cage line and never beyond. In the closed position, the echo line from the cage is recorded halfway between the cage and sewing ring in an almost parallel position.

  Reverberations are seen below the valve tracings representing echo reflections from the posterior surface of the ball.

- A St Jude valve in the open position shows parallel lines of the disc parallel to the sewing ring. In the closed position, no echo lines are recorded (the disc lies within the sewing ring).

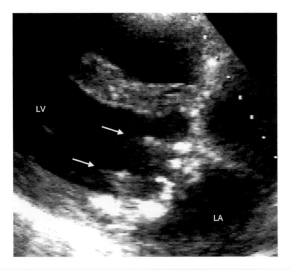

Fig. 6.6 *Mitral valve biological prosthetic valve. Parasternal long-axis view showing the normal appearance of 2 of the supporting stents (arrows) within the left ventricular cavity.*

- In biological prostheses, the sewing ring is seen as a continuous echo line. Leaflets show echo tracings similar to native valves, with a leaflet excursion giving a box-like shape. Echo lines representing 2 of the 3 stents may be seen.

2-D echo gives important anatomical information. If no surgical operative details are available, some aspects of the echo examination may help to identify which sort of valve is present (it is easier to make this assessment for mitral (Fig. 6.6) than aortic valves):

- Ball and cage – characteristic semicircular echo image of the cage with the ball moving up and down
- Tilting disc – the movement of one or two discs can be seen opening and closing
- Tissue – the metal stents can often be seen in the LV cavity (mitral) or aorta (aortic).

Doppler echo is very useful in evaluating prosthetic valve function:

Obstruction to flow

Because of the non-compliant nature of the material in these valves, velocity of flow through them has a different range from normal native valves. Most prosthetic valves give some obstruction to flow. A number of measurements can be made:

1. *Peak velocity.* This is higher than in normal valves because of the relatively smaller orifice area caused by the bulk of the artificial material. An example of the range is given below.

   As a general rule of thumb, a peak velocity of >2 m/s in the MV usually indicates dysfunction in both mechanical and biological prosthetic valves. Aortic prosthesis flow velocity is normally <3 m/s.

2. *Pressure gradient* (ΔP). This is calculated by the simplified Bernoulli equation ($\Delta P = 4V^2$).

3. *Valve orifice area* – is measured using the continuity equation (Ch. 3).

Different echo labs have different ranges. A change in velocity from postoperative values is more important in an individual case.

Regurgitation

This may be through the valve orifice (transvalvular) or around the sewing ring (paraprosthetic). Mild transvalvular MR can be found in normally functioning

Velocity of flow (m/s) through some normally-functioning mechanical and tissue prosthetic valves		
Valve	**Mitral**	**Aortic**
Ball and cage Starr–Edwards	1.4–2.2	2.6–3.0
Single disc Björk–Shiley	1.3–1.8	1.9–2.9
Double disc St Jude	1.2–1.8	2.3–2.8
Porcine biological Carpentier–Edwards	1.5–2.0	1.9–2.8

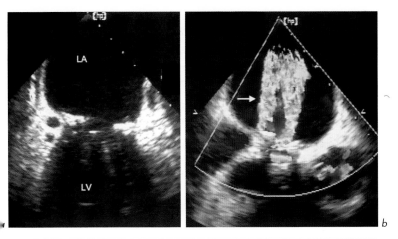

Fig. 6.7 *Regurgitation through a Starr–Edwards mitral valve prosthesis. Two jets can be seen on colour flow Doppler – a transvalvular jet and a paraprosthetic jet (arrow).*

valves, more often in mechanical valves. This is due to valve closure or through the gaps between different parts of the prosthesis. It can be difficult to detect this due to masking. Moderate or severe MR is abnormal.

Continuous wave Doppler is more useful than pulsed wave and colour flow is good for showing anterograde and retrograde flows. Turbulent forward flow is shown as a mosaic of colours. In mitral bioprostheses one jet is usually seen. In most mitral mechanical valves, 2 jets are seen (almost equal size in Starr–Edwards, one smaller than the other in Björk–Shiley valves).

In regurgitation (Fig. 6.7), there may be a number of jets of different sizes depending on valve type (e.g. 2 jets in Björk–Shiley, multiple in Starr–Edwards). Colour flow also helps in differentiating between transvalvular and paravalvular regurgitation and helps to show new regurgitation.

Prosthetic valve malfunction

A false diagnosis of malfunction may be made if there is a low cardiac output, arrhythmia such as AV block or poor surgical technique (e.g. valve which is too small or too large for the heart). Types of malfunction include:

- In mechanical and biological valves: endocarditis, dehiscence (valve becomes loose or detached), regurgitation
- More common in mechanical valves: thrombus, variance (change in shape or size)
- More common in biological valves: degeneration – stenosis or regurgitation.

Echo features of valve malfunction

Findings should be compared with baseline values where possible.

1. Anatomical abnormalities of prosthesis (by M-mode and 2-D echo):
    - Loose part of valve, e.g. ruptured bioprosthesis leaflet
    - Loose sutures
    - Abnormal motion – reduced or exaggerated motion of any part of prosthesis
    - Associated findings, e.g. calcification, thrombus, vegetation, abscess, increased chamber size (LV, LA).
2. Haemodynamic abnormalities of prosthesis (by Doppler and colour flow):
    - Obstruction may be suggested by increased flow velocity or reduced orifice area
    - Regurgitation – increased severity of jet or new jet.

Endocarditis of prosthetic valves

This is a very serious problem and often results in a need for the valve to be surgically replaced, often after a period of treatment with i.v. antibiotics. Antibiotic prophylaxis for all dental treatment and surgery is essential to try to prevent this. Endocarditis can affect mechanical or biological prostheses. It occurs at an annual rate of 3–5% in those with prosthetic valves.

The following are suggestive findings:

- Vegetations (mobile masses on valve, move in cardiac cycle, but are often hard to see)
- Incomplete valve closure due to interference by vegetations with valve leaflets
- Abscess seen as poorly echo-reflective areas around sewing ring
- Sutures may be seen moving freely if dehiscence occurs.

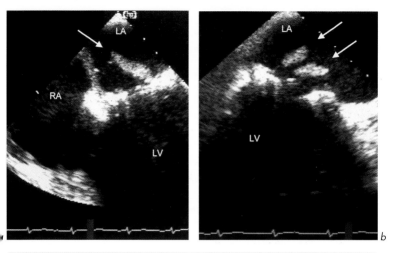

Fig. 6.8 (a) and *(b)* Large vegetations (arrows) seen on the atrial side of a Starr–Edwards mitral valve prosthesis.

M-mode may show vegetations as multiple thick echo lines superimposed on M-mode of prosthesis, but both **M-mode** and **2-D echo** may be difficult because of reverberations and masking. Small vegetations (<2–3 mm) may be missed. It can be difficult sometimes to distinguish vegetations from calcified or thickened leaflets.

Doppler and **colour flow** can show haemodynamic consequences of endocarditis – transvalvular regurgitation (vegetations affecting leaflet closure), paravalvular regurgitation (abscess formation at suture lines), or increased forward flow due to obstruction by vegetation. As mentioned, TOE is very useful in these situations (Fig. 6.8).

Thrombus

More common in mechanical valves and responsible for many cases of malfunction. This can occur if anticoagulation control is poor or in the presence of dilated cardiac chambers.

Anticoagulation is essential for all mechanical valves (aim for international normalized ratio (INR) of 3.5–5.0). Prosthetic valves' susceptibility to thrombosis depends on their position (related to the pressure gradient across the valve):

tricuspid > mitral > pulmonary > aortic.

Sometimes, patients complain that they can no longer hear the valve clicking – this may be an indication of thrombosis.

Echo can detect thrombus by:

- Visualization of a mobile mass on the valve – it can be hard to distinguish from vegetations or calcified nodules
- Reduced or absent motion of the mobile part of the valve, e.g. ball, disc, cusps
- Associated dilatation of cardiac chambers.

As with vegetations, **M-mode** may show multiple dark echo lines and/or reduced valve opening or closing. **Doppler** and **colour flow** may show obstruction of valve opening (increased flow velocity) or obstruction of closure (a new transvalvular regurgitant jet or increase in severity of existing regurgitation).

Dehiscence

This is the failure of the sutures to attach the valve ring to the surrounding native tissues because of either loosening or rupture of one or more sutures. This may result in paravalvular regurgitation and/or abnormal valve motion (e.g. valve rocking or sutures may be seen moving freely).

Regurgitation

Transvalvular. A mild degree is often seen as part of the normal function of the valve. It is increased by any factor that causes incomplete closure of prosthetic valves, e.g. vegetation, thrombus, variance or degeneration. It can be detected by colour flow or continuous wave Doppler.

Paravalvular. This is abnormal. It can be caused by endocarditis (abscess), dehiscence or other causes. Colour flow will show a regurgitant jet through an area outside the sewing ring.

Variance

This is less common with the newer mechanical valves. It is a change in the shape and size of a mechanical valve due to erosions or cracks in the body of the ball or the disc or deposition of material into the valve (e.g. fibrous tissue or lipids onto the ball or metallic surface of the prosthesis).

The ball or disc becomes larger or smaller causing obstruction or incomplete closure, respectively. Echo can detect reduced motion of the ball or disc, increased flow velocity or transvalvular regurgitation.

Degeneration

Degeneration occurs in most biological prostheses within a few years. This leads to calcification and stenosis and/or rupture of valve leaflets and regurgitation towards the end of the expected lifespan of the valve. Echo may show calcification, abnormal leaflet motion and/or regurgitation.

6.4 CONGENITAL ABNORMALITIES

Echo is essential in the diagnosis of congenital heart disease and has reduced the need for cardiac catheterization in such conditions. Echo allows anatomical and haemodynamic assessment (e.g. the location and size of shunts, cardiac chamber anatomy and connections, and pressures such as pulmonary artery pressure).

1. Shunts

The term 'cardiac shunt' describes the flow of blood through an abnormal communication between different cardiac chambers or blood vessels. Examples of such communications are ASD, VSD or PDA. Blood will flow from a region of higher pressure to a region of lower pressure, usually left to right (e.g. LV to RV across a VSD). This results in increased blood flow and raised pressures on the right heart. Untreated, this can lead to right heart dilatation and failure. In some cases, irreversible changes in the pulmonary vasculature occur and the resistance in these vessels increases. This raises right-sided pressures with PHT (**Eisenmenger reaction** – the combination of a shunt with PHT) which may exceed left-sided pressures. 'Shunt reversal' then occurs (right to left shunting). This causes central cyanosis as deoxygenated blood enters the systemic circulation.

The larger the size of the shunt (the more blood passing across an abnormal communication), the more likely it is to be haemodynamically significant and require closure of the defect. Note that when the Eisenmenger reaction has occurred it is usually too late to close a defect safely, since right heart failure may occur and is often fatal.

VSD, ASD, PFO (Figs 6.9, 6.10, 6.11)

Defects may be identified in the ventricular or atrial septa by 2-D studies. The direction of flow across such defects can be shown by colour flow mapping and the velocity of the jet across the defect can be measured (and hence the pressure gradient identified) by continuous wave Doppler. This is especially useful in VSDs where a high velocity jet suggests a high-pressure gradient between LV and RV and is referred to as a restrictive VSD. This is less likely to have a large shunt. VSD can occur in the upper membranous or lower muscular septum.

The interatrial septum (IAS) is often thin and in certain views in normal individuals (especially the apical 4-chamber view) there can appear to be a defect in a normal septum, giving the false illusion of an ASD. This is due to an effect

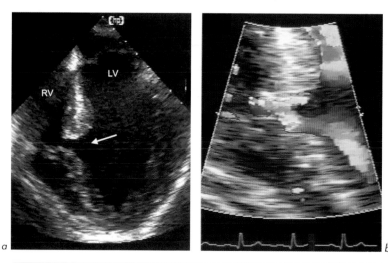

a   *b*

Fig. 6.9 (a) *Muscular ventricular septal defect (arrow).* (b) *Colour flow mapping shows flow from left to right ventricle.*

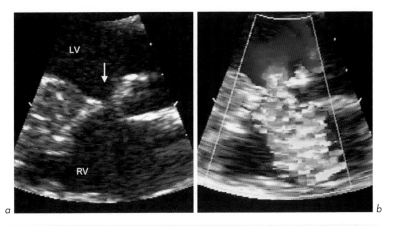

Fig. 6.10 (a) *Membranous ventricular septal defect (arrow).* **(b)** *Colour flow from left to right ventricle.*

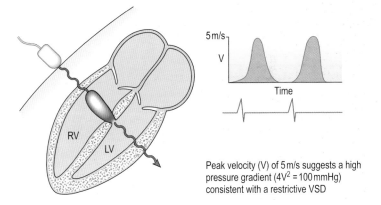

Peak velocity (V) of 5 m/s suggests a high pressure gradient (4V² = 100 mmHg) consistent with a restrictive VSD

Fig. 6.11 *Continuous wave Doppler showing high velocity flow across a ventricular septal defect from left to right ventricle.*

known as 'echo drop-out' which happens because the reflected echo signal from the IAS is weak. The IAS in this view is being hit along its edge by the ultrasound beam and is at a large depth from the transducer. By examining the IAS from other views (e.g. subcostal), it can be seen that it is intact.

TOE allows excellent visualization of IAS and hence diagnosis of ASD (Figs 6.12, 6.13) and PFO. It can detect the size, number and type (location) of ASD,

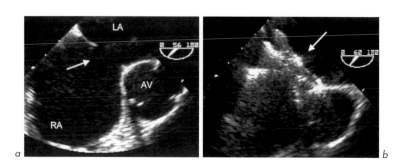

Fig. 6.12 (a) Ostium secundum atrial septal defect (arrow). (b) Following percutaneous closure with Amplatz device (arrow). Note the acoustic shadow cast by the device and seen in the right atrium on TOE.

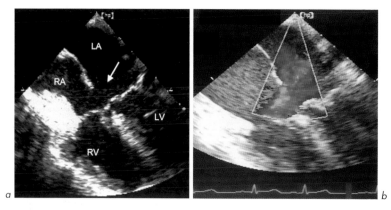

Fig. 6.13 (a) Ostium primum atrial sepal defect (arrow) on TOE 4-chamber view. (b) Colour flow mapping demonstrating flow across the defect.

and suitability for percutaneous catheter-guided device closure rather than surgery.

Currently, **device closure for ASD** is suitable if:

- Not multiple
- Not too close to MV or TV
- Size <30 mm.

TTE and TOE are both good at diagnosing ostium primum ASDs but TOE is better than TTE in diagnosing secundum ASDs under 10 mm diameter. Defects of under 5 mm are only diagnosed correctly by TTE 20% of the time. 5–10 mm secundum ASDs are detected by TTE in 80% of cases.

Most clinically and haemodynamically significant ASDs should be diagnosed by TTE. However, TOE should be considered where left-to-right shunting is suspected but not proven on TTE (even after contrast study) or where a small defect may be significant, e.g. after trans-septal puncture at catheterization. TOE is superior at identifying associated abnormalities, e.g. partial anomalous pulmonary venous drainage.

PFO is seen in up to 30% at autopsy. TTE and TOE contrast studies show a prevalence of 10–35%. TOE colour flow mapping detects only one-third of those shown on contrast injection – for this reason, a contrast study should always be performed if a shunt is suspected.

Device closure for PFO may be considered in individuals who:

- Have suffered a stroke thought to be due to paradoxical (right-to-left) embolization across the PFO
- Suffer from migraine. Studies are still underway to determine whether this technique is an effective treatment in migraine.

Bubble/contrast studies (Fig. 6.14)

Contrast studies are often useful in determining whether there is flow across the IAS. This can be done with commercially available contrast agents or with saline which has a small amount of the patient's blood or air bubbles agitated in a syringe. This is injected into a peripheral vein, and contrast is seen in the RA and then the RV. The subject is often asked to perform a Valsalva manoeuvre to increase intrathoracic pressure. Contrast may be seen shunting from RA to LA in the presence of an ASD or PFO, or RV to LV in the presence of a VSD. A bubble contrast study may be positive even when no obvious flow is detected on colour flow mapping.

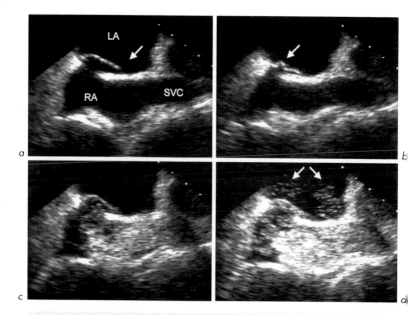

Fig. 6.14 Patent foramen ovale (PFO) and bubble contrast TOE study. **(a)** The PFO is shown (arrow). **(b)** 'Buckling' of the interatrial septum (arrow). **(c)** Bubble contrast reaches right atrium. **(d)** Some bubbles are seen to cross the PFO from right to left atrium (arrows).

Indications for bubble/contrast echo study include:
- Suspected ASD, VSD or PFO
- Dilated RA and/or dilated RV of unknown cause
- PHT of unknown cause.

Patent ductus arteriosus

This is a condition in which the ductus arteriosus remains open after birth. This provides a communication between the aorta and PA. A continuous murmur occurs in systole and diastole (a 'machinery' murmur). Echo can be used to detect the presence of the shunt and give an estimate of its haemodynamic significance.

Eisenmenger reaction

This occurs when an intracardiac or extracardiac shunt is associated with PHT. Echo is very important in providing noninvasive assessment allowing the underlying cause to be seen (e.g. VSD), estimating the PASP by the peak Doppler velocity of TR and assessing complications such as severity of TR and size and function of the RV.

2. Coarctation of the aorta

Coarctation (narrowing) of the aorta may be detected using echo and the peak velocity across the coarctation (and hence the pressure gradient) can be measured. This is usually achieved using continuous wave Doppler with the transducer in the suprasternal notch (Fig. 6.15).

3. Congenital valvular abnormalities

Bicuspid aortic valve (Fig. 6.16)

This is the commonest congenital cardiac abnormality (1–2% of the population). This can be seen by its features on M-mode echo (eccentric closure line) and on

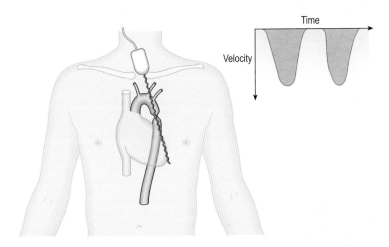

Fig. 6.15 *Examination of a coarctation of the thoracic aorta by continuous wave Doppler with the transducer in the suprasternal notch.*

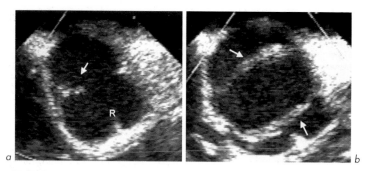

Fig. 6.16 *Bicuspid aortic valve – TOE short-axis study. (a) Closed valve showing eccentric closure line (arrow) and median raphe (R) representing the region where 2 leaflets are congenitally fused. (b) Open valve showing 2 leaflets (arrows).*

2-D echo, particularly in parasternal short-axis view at aortic level. It may occur in isolation or in association with other congenital conditions (e.g. coarctation). It may cause AS. Other abnormalities of the AV may be detected (e.g. 4-leaflet valve – very rare! (Fig. 6.17)).

Ebstein's anomaly (Figs 6.18, 6.19)

A rare but important group of abnormalities. The characteristic feature of this is tricuspid valve dysplasia (malformation) with downward (apical) displacement of the TV into the body of the RV. There is consequent 'atrialization' of the upper part of the RV. Abnormalities of the TV leaflets and chordae include tricuspid atresia (absent development), and can cause TS or TR. 2-D and Doppler echo can show the abnormality present and its consequences.

Pulmonary stenosis

This may occur as a congenital abnormality and even quite high degrees of obstruction can be tolerated into adult life (particularly if RV function is good, there is no associated severe TR and sinus rhythm is maintained). It may be valvular or due to narrowing in the pulmonary artery or RV outflow tract. Continuous wave Doppler and 2-D echo can assess severity, the effect upon RV size and function, associated congenital lesions and the presence and severity of TR.

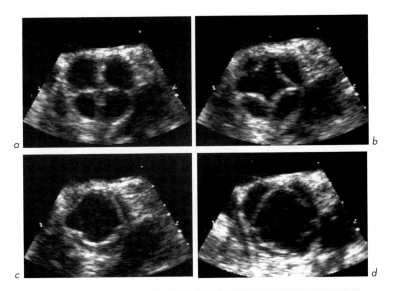

Fig. 6.17 *Four-cusp aortic valve. The valve is shown in closed position and at various stages of opening. The anatomy was confirmed at surgery for severe aortic regurgitation. This congenital abnormality is very rare.*

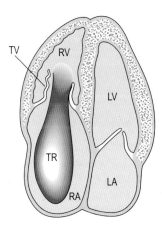

Fig. 6.18 *Ebstein's anomaly. Apical displacement of tricuspid valve (TV) which is often malformed causing tricuspid stenosis or severe regurgitation as shown.*

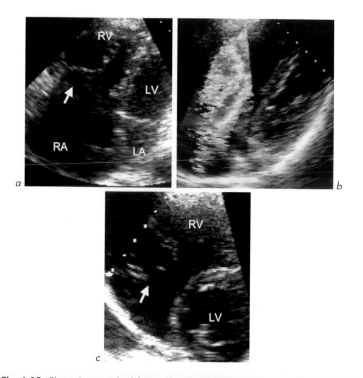

Fig. 6.19 *Ebstein's anomaly.* **(a)** *Apical 4-chamber view showing malformation of the tricuspid valve (arrow).* **(b)** *Colour flow mapping showing severe tricuspid regurgitation.* **(c)** *Parasternal short-axis view showing dilated right ventricle and malformed tricuspid valve (arrow).*

4. Complex congenital abnormalities

These are beyond the scope of this book, but one condition is worth mentioning: **tetralogy of Fallot** (Figs 6.20, 6.21) – characterized by:

1. VSD – usually perimembranous
2. Overriding aorta – displaced to the right and loss of continuity with IVS
3. RV outflow tract obstruction (RVOTO) – at different sites, often in combination – infundibular (subvalvular) in 70–80%, valvular in 20–40%. Supravalvular is less common
4. RV hypertrophy.

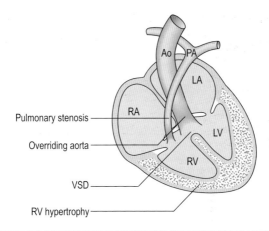

Pulmonary stenosis

Overriding aorta

VSD

RV hypertrophy

Fig. 6.20 Tetralogy of Fallot.

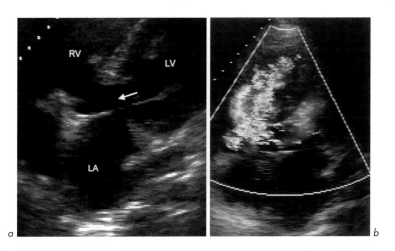

a

b

Fig. 6.21 Tetralogy of Fallot. Colour flow through the ventricular septal defect (arrow) on apical 4-chamber view.

Echo can help in diagnosis of tetralogy of Fallot, nowadays usually in infancy, and in follow-up after surgical repair to examine adequacy of VSD closure, residual RVOTO, severity of PR and RV thickness and function.

5. Echo method to estimate cardiac output and shunt size

Echo can give an estimate of the size of a shunt. The method is simple but requires some explanation. One first needs to understand how echo can give an estimate of cardiac output from the left heart:

$$\text{Cardiac output} = \text{stroke volume} \times \text{heart rate}$$

Stroke volume is derived by echo from a measure known as the 'flow velocity integral' (FVI) (Fig. 6.22). This is calculated by the computer of the echo machine as the area under the curve from the continuous wave Doppler of aortic outflow in the apical 5-chamber view. FVI is given from peak aortic flow velocity, V_{max} in cm/s and aortic ejection time in seconds/beat:

$$\text{Stroke volume} = \text{FVI} \times \text{cross-sectional area (of aortic valve)}$$

$$\text{Cross-sectional area (CSA)} = \pi r^2 = \pi(D/2)^2 = 3.14D^2/4 \approx 0.75D^2$$

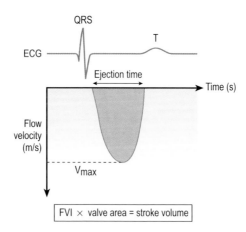

Fig. 6.22 *Flow velocity integral (FVI) of aortic flow (shaded area).*

where D is AV diameter measured either from M-mode of the AV tracing or from the parasternal long-axis view measured in the aortic root just above the tips of the aortic cusps.

Normal values in adults at rest:

- Stroke volume   70–140 mL/beat
- Cardiac output   4–7 L/min
- Cardiac index*   2.8–4.2 L/min/m^2
  (* cardiac index is cardiac output corrected for BSA).

Now a similar method is applied to the right heart (to measure pulmonary flow, Qp) as for the left heart (to measure aortic or systemic flow, Qs). The size of a shunt in an ASD or VSD can be estimated from the ratio of the pulmonary to the aortic flow. This ratio is Qp/Qs.

As a rough guide, a shunt is haemodynamically significant if the shunt ratio (Qp/Qs) is >2.0.

$$Q_P/Q_S = \frac{FVI_{pulmonary} \times D^2_{pulmonary}}{FVI_{aortic} \times D^2_{aortic}}$$

- $FVI_{pulmonary}$ is calculated from the Doppler signal of pulmonary systolic flow from the parasternal short-axis view at aortic level.
- $D_{pulmonary}$ is the PV diameter obtained in the same view at the base of the PV leaflets.

CHAPTER 7

Special situations and conditions

7.1 PREGNANCY

Echo in pregnancy is safe. Many pregnant women develop systolic murmurs due to increased cardiac output (which rises by 30–50% in pregnancy). Many murmurs are benign (e.g. mammary souffle) but some may not be. Cardiac disease can present and be diagnosed for the first time during pregnancy, or those with pre-existing heart disease may become pregnant and may suffer deterioration in their cardiac state. Echo is essential in both situations. Some may suffer troublesome palpitations and whilst this is a less clear-cut indication for echo, the finding of normal LV function, chamber size and valve function can be very reassuring.

Anatomical and echo changes in pregnancy can include:
- Mild increases in cardiac chamber size including RA and RV. LA increases by 10–15% and LV by 5–10%.
- Increased stroke volume (increased flow velocity integral of AV and PV).
- Small pericardial effusions (20%) causing no haemodynamic compromise. If there is compromise, another cause must be sought.
- Peripartum cardiomyopathy.
- Vascular 'laxity' in peripartum period. Both aortic and coronary artery spontaneous dissections are more common, but still rare.
- In late pregnancy, the enlarged uterus may increase intra-abdominal pressure causing compression of the thoracic structures and a pseudo-posterior wall motion abnormality as occurs in liver disease with ascites.

Of course, there are a number of congenital cardiac abnormalities that have important implications for pregnancy.

The body of knowledge relating to high cardiac-risk pregnancies is increasing. Many women with such pregnancies are managed in specialized centres where a multidisciplinary team including obstetricians, midwives, cardiologists, anaesthetists, nurses and cardiac technicians work together to minimize the risks. Echo often plays an important part in the decision-making process.

1. Cardiac lesions associated with high risk (to mother)

- PHT (primary or secondary to Eisenmenger)
- AS
- MS
- Marfan's syndrome
- HCM (especially if high degree of outflow tract obstruction)
- Any lesion causing New York Heart Association grade 4 breathlessness (i.e. at rest or on minimal exertion).

Eisenmenger's reaction (PHT with a shunt) carries a high maternal (30–70%) and fetal mortality. Maternal mortality is due to arrhythmia, increased cyanosis, low cardiac output, catastrophic rise in PA pressure and right heart failure. The early postpartum period is particularly dangerous, possibly related to sudden alterations in venous return.

In AS or MS, pregnancy increases the valve gradient as cardiac output rises and systemic vascular resistance falls. MS can be very difficult in pregnancy. Echo allows noninvasive assessment of valve orifice and PA pressures and may help to determine timing of delivery or valvotomy.

In Marfan's syndrome, the dominant hazard is aortic root dilatation and aortic dissection made more likely by haemodynamic changes and weakening of the aortic wall by hormonal changes.

Echo allows serial noninvasive assessment of PASP during pregnancy when this is elevated (e.g. primary or secondary to MV disease or Eisenmenger's).

2. Intermediate (moderate) risk lesions

- Coarctation
- Cyanotic heart disease without PHT
- Prosthetic valves – risks are of premature valve failure (biological prostheses), thromboembolism, complications related to warfarin/heparin (e.g. teratogenesis, fetal growth retardation, placental haemorrhage, osteoporosis)
- Tetralogy of Fallot – can behave unpredictably – increased venous return and systemic vasodilatation can cause profound hypoxia.

3. Lower-risk lesions are fortunately the most common

- Uncomplicated ASD or VSD, although there is a risk of paradoxical embolization. One particular problem of unoperated ASD or VSD occurs at delivery. Blood loss may lower RA pressure and increase left to right shunting, stealing from the systemic circulation, sometimes progressively and catastrophically. Intravenous fluid replacement must be rigorous in these patients.
- MR, AR and PS are usually well tolerated in pregnancy.

Benign maternal murmurs in pregnancy (see section 1.6)

- Pulmonary flow murmur – at left sternal edge at 2nd intercostal space. Due to increased cardiac output and flow into the pulmonary circulation
- Venous hum
- Mammary souffle – associated with lactation and ceasing when that ends.

Peripartum cardiomyopathy

Echo shows a dilated LV with impaired systolic function. It presents in the later part of pregnancy and in the postpartum months. The echo features are identical to those of dilated cardiomyopathy. It may represent pre-existing dilated cardiomyopathy undiagnosed before pregnancy. The prognosis relates to the severity of heart failure and how rapidly cardiac size returns to normal. If present for more than 6 months, the prognosis is poor. Treatment is conventional (diuretics and ACE inhibitors). It may recur in subsequent pregnancies.

Fetal welfare

The risks mentioned relate to the mother. Fetal welfare must of course be assessed during these pregnancies. The hazards to the fetus relate to:

1. Maternal cyanosis
2. Need for bypass surgery during pregnancy (20% risk of fetal loss)
3. Drug therapy:
   - Warfarin – fetal haemorrhage and multiple congenital abnormalities
   - Heparin – retroplacental haemorrhage
   - ACE inhibitors – neonatal renal failure, oligohydramnios, growth retardation
   - β-blockers – intrauterine growth restriction, neonatal hypoglycaemia, bradycardia

4. Genetic risk of transmission
   - Marfan's syndrome, HCM and other single gene defects – 50%
   - Multifactorial conditions such as ASD or VSD – transmission rate 4–6%, compared with prevalence in the general population of 1%.

Fetal echo

Fetal echo (by transabdominal or transvaginal ultrasound examination) is carried out in a number of specialist centres to determine if there is a cardiac abnormality in the unborn child. Some cases have been surgically corrected *in utero*.

7.2 RHYTHM DISTURBANCES

Arrhythmias can be primary abnormalities or occur in association with structural heart disease. This may include congenital abnormalities or those of the myocardium, valves, pericardium or coronary arteries. The main use of echo is in determining associated heart disease.

Atrial fibrillation (AF) or flutter

Fibrillation refers to the situation when electrical activity is not coordinated in a chamber and individual muscle fibres contract independently. This can occur in atrial or ventricular muscle. Ventricular fibrillation (VF), unless promptly terminated, is fatal. AF can be tolerated, and, apart from the occurrence of atrial and ventricular extrasystoles, is the most common arrhythmia in many countries. An underlying cause for AF should always be sought.

Common causes of AF

- Ischaemic heart disease
- Rheumatic heart disease, e.g. MS
- Hypertension
- Toxins, e.g. ethanol
- Thyroid disease – usually thyrotoxicosis
- Infection – myocarditis, pneumonia
- Myocardial disease, e.g. dilated cardiomyopathy
- Lung disease
- Pulmonary embolism

- Pericardial disease, e.g. pericarditis
- 'Lone' – no underlying cause found.

All individuals with AF should have an echo. This is to determine an underlying cause (e.g. MS), assess the risk of complications (such as stroke, see below) and assess the likelihood of successful restoration to normal sinus rhythm (cardioversion) by electrical or chemical means.

Echo detects an underlying cardiac disorder in approximately 10% of subjects with AF who have no other clinically suspected heart disease and in 60% of those with some indicators of heart disease.

Restoration of sinus rhythm is *less* likely to be successful if there is:

- MV disease
- An enlarged LA
- LV dysfunction
- Thyroid disease
- Long-standing AF.

Unless there is a contraindication, individuals with AF have an improved prognosis if treated with anticoagulants such as warfarin. This is certainly true for rheumatic AF and probably in non-rheumatic AF where there is an underlying cause. It is less certain in 'lone' AF. This benefit increases with the age of the individual.

The annual risk of stroke is increased in subjects with LA enlargement or LV dysfunction:

Findings	Annual stroke risk (%)
Normal heart – sinus rhythm	0.3
'Lone' AF	0.5
AF with normal echo	1.5
AF with enlarged LA >2.5 cm/m^2	8.8
AF with global LV dysfunction	12.6
AF with enlarged LA (>2.5 cm/m^2) and moderate LV dysfunction	20.0

Data from Stroke Prevention in Atrial Fibrillation Study Group Investigators. *Ann Intern Med* 1992; 116:6–12.

There is evidence to suggest that, in many individuals with AF, heart rate control (e.g. with digoxin, β-blockers or calcium-channel blockers) and long-term anticoagulation with warfarin is preferable to attempting rhythm control (i.e. cardioversion). Cardioversion may be considered if:

- Recent-onset AF with an identifiable reversible cause (e.g. recent treated pneumonia)
- Subject is very symptomatic and unable to tolerate AF and/or rate-controlling medications
- AF has caused heart failure
- Individual is unable to take long-term anticoagulants.

Following successful cardioversion, warfarin should be continued for 3–6 months, since the return of atrial mechanical activity (at which time thromboembolism might occur) is often delayed, due to atrial 'stunning', relative to the restoration of synchronized atrial electrical activity.

In some individuals with AF, catheter ablation of the rhythm disturbance is considered.

Echo before cardioversion

This may help to identify those most likely to have successful cardioversion to sinus rhythm or to predict those at increased risk of thromboembolic complications. Previous data suggest that 5–7% of subjects undergoing cardioversion who have not been anticoagulated suffer thromboembolic complications. These may not occur until some time after cardioversion. The most likely explanation is that atrial mechanical activity may not return for some time after the restoration of atrial electrical activity.

There is some controversy regarding the use of TOE in patients with chronic AF (>48 h) prior to cardioversion. Pre- and post-cardioversion anticoagulation is indicated and large studies are underway. There is less information in recent-onset AF (<48 h) but present data suggest that 14% of patients with recent AF have LA appendage thrombus, suggesting that these patients should also be anticoagulated.

Indications for TOE before cardioversion

- Urgent cardioversion needed when pre-cardioversion anticoagulation not possible
- Prior thromboembolic events thought to be related to LA thrombus

- Previous demonstration of LA thrombus
- If finding co-existent factors influences decision to cardiovert (e.g. LV function, MV disease)
- AF of <48 h
- AF in the presence of MV disease or HCM, even if anticoagulated.

Ventricular tachycardia (VT) or fibrillation (VF)

These are important indications for echo. The underlying cause is often coronary artery disease, and there may be features of ischaemia and/or infarction. VT of LV origin is frequently associated with reduced LV function. It may complicate an underlying cardiomyopathy (e.g. dilated or hypertrophic). VT of RV origin may suggest an RV structural abnormality such as RV dysplasia.

Syncope

This means sudden loss of consciousness. It can have a number of neurological or cardiac causes. The role of echo relates to its ability to detect obstructive lesions (e.g. AS, HCM) or abnormalities such as LV impairment that may be associated with arrhythmias such as VT. The use of echo routinely in syncopal subjects is controversial.

Indications include:
- Syncope with suspected heart disease
- Exertional syncope
- Syncope in high-risk occupation (e.g. pilot).

Palpitations

Many individuals experience atrial or ventricular ectopic beats. The indication for echo in these cases is less clear-cut. An echo should be carried out if there is any suspicion of structural heart disease (abnormality on history, e.g. associated symptoms such as syncope, clinical examination, ECG or chest X-ray). Otherwise the pick-up rate is very low. A normal echo (normal LV, other chambers and valves) can be reassuring for an anxious individual.

In general, echo does not need to be performed in a subject with palpitations for which an arrhythmic cause has been ruled out.

7.3 HYPERTENSION AND LVH (Fig. 7.1)

Main indications for echo in hypertension

- Assessment of LV systolic and diastolic function
- Detection of LVH and response to treatment
- Detection/effects of co-existing coronary disease (e.g. by stress echo)
- Possible underlying cause of hypertension (e.g. aortic coarctation).

Hypertension is the most important cause of LVH, which is an independent predictive factor for cardiovascular mortality and morbidity. It predicts the risk of MI, heart failure or sudden cardiac death and is as predictive as the occurrence of multi-vessel coronary artery disease. LVH may be indicated on voltage criteria on ECG recording (large voltage QRS complexes) The criteria differ but S in V1 or V2 plus R in V5 or V6 > 35 mm is useful (Sokolow criteria). Some subjects with thin chest walls may have voltage criteria for LVH on ECG but normal LV wall thickness. There may be associated 'strain pattern' on ECG in LVH (ST segment depression and T-wave inversion in the lateral leads).

Echo allows wall thickness to be measured accurately and is more sensitive than ECG at detecting LVH. The presence of LVH can help to determine if

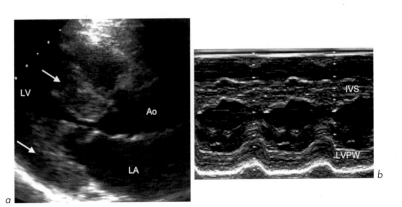

Fig. 7.1 *Severe concentric left ventricular hypertrophy in long-standing hypertension. (a) Parasternal long-axis view showing left ventricular hypertrophy of septum and posterior wall (arrows). (b) M-mode.*

treatment is necessary in subjects with borderline hypertension. Echo can also be used to assess whether there is regression of LVH with antihypertensive treatment.

LVH is often considered present if the IVS or LVPW thickness is above 'normal limits' (often >12 mm in diastole). Strictly speaking, one should measure LV mass to diagnose LVH. This can be calculated from M-mode or 2-D measurements of IVS and LVPW thickness in diastole and LVEDD, all in cm, by an equation suggested by Devereux and Reichek (*Circulation* 1977; 55: 613–618):

$$LV\ mass(g) \simeq 1.04\,[(LVEDD + IVS + LVPW)^3 - LVEDD^3] - 14$$

This should be corrected for height or BSA (which gives 'LV mass index'). The 'normal values' are:

	Women	Men
LV mass corrected for height (g/m)	89 ± 25	114 ± 35
LV mass corrected for BSA ('LV mass index') (g/m²)	112	136

7.4 STROKE, TIA AND THROMBOEMBOLISM

'Is there a cardiac source of embolism?'

This is a fairly common question asked when an echo is requested. It can be quite difficult to answer, particularly by TTE. TOE may provide more information.

Ultrasound examination of patients with stroke or TIA in territories outside the vertebrobasilar territories is certainly important but echo is not the only useful test. Ultrasound scanning of the carotid arteries may provide useful diagnostic information and finding significant carotid stenosis (>70%) is an indication for carotid endarterectomy.

In the presence of a normal cardiovascular history, examination and ECG, the likelihood of a TTE detecting a cardiac abnormality in stroke or TIA is very low.

The main purposes of echo are:

- To make a diagnosis associated with risk of thromboembolism (e.g. MS, LV dilatation)

- To detect a direct source of embolism from an intracardiac mass – thrombus, tumour, vegetation.

Indications for echo in stroke, TIA or vascular occlusive events

- Sudden occlusion of a peripheral or visceral artery
- Younger patients (<50 years) with stroke or TIA
- Older patients (>50 years) with stroke or TIA without evidence of cerebrovascular disease or other obvious cause
- Suspicion of embolic disease
- Clinical evidence of cardiac abnormality, e.g. abnormal physical signs (murmur, suspected endocarditis) or abnormal ECG (MI, arrhythmia such as AF, VT or nonspecific ST-T abnormalities).

TOE may be indicated (with a normal or inconclusive TTE) if:

- High suspicion of embolism (e.g. endocarditis)
- Young patient (many centres arbitrarily say age <50 years).

The risk of thromboembolism is so high in MS, particularly if AF is present, that anticoagulation should be considered if there is no contraindication and cerebral haemorrhage has been excluded by CT scanning. This is true even if the echo does not show obvious thrombus (remember, LA thrombus is often not seen on TTE). Alternatively, echo may show a large LA ball thrombus which is an indication for urgent surgery.

In young subjects, it is generally agreed that TTE and TOE should be carried out to look for treatable rare causes of stroke such as:

- Left atrial myxoma (which has been estimated to occur in 1% of such cases)
- LA spontaneous contrast
- LA appendage thrombus
- PFO (venous thrombus can 'paradoxically' embolize from right to left)
- Aneurysm of IAS (increased risk of thromboembolism possibly due to frequent association with PFO)
- Aortic atheroma.

7.5 BREATHLESSNESS AND PERIPHERAL OEDEMA

Breathlessness is an important symptom of many heart diseases. In the presence of heart failure, it usually indicates pulmonary venous hypertension. The causes of breathlessness are numerous. Cardiac diseases often co-exist with respiratory causes such as chronic airflow limitation.

Echo is an essential test in a breathless patient where the history, examination and routine tests such as ECG and chest X-ray suggest or cannot exclude heart disease. It may reveal:

- LV systolic and/or diastolic dysfunction
- Left-sided valve disease
- Cardiomyopathy.

Oedema has a number of cardiac and non-cardiac causes. The cardiac causes are any conditions that increase the central venous pressure and include myocardial, pericardial and valvular abnormalities. Echo is useful in these cases. In cases of peripheral oedema with a normal JVP, echo is *not* likely to be helpful (unless the patient has been receiving treatment with diuretics).

Other causes of oedema should be investigated:

- Renal failure
- Protein-losing states, e.g. nephrotic syndrome
- Hypoalbuminaemia, e.g. liver disease
- Deep venous thrombosis
- Venous incompetence
- Pelvic obstruction
- Endocrine abnormality, e.g. hypothyroidism.

7.6 SCREENING AND FOLLOW-UP ECHO

Who should have a screening echo?

If screening asymptomatic individuals, some criteria should be met:

- The test should be safe, accurate, readily available and inexpensive – echo satisfies these.
- The abnormality should have a reasonable frequency to allow detection.
- Detection should alter management or provide prognostic information.

There are no clear-cut rules. Some suggestions:

Good indications for screening echo

1. Individuals with a family history of genetically transmitted cardiovascular disease:

- First-degree relatives of sufferers of HCM – many screen every 5 years from age 5 up to age 20 (if normal by that age, the diagnosis is excluded). Approximately 1 in 5 first-degree relatives of individuals with HCM were found to have the condition in a large-scale screening study.
- Suspected collagen abnormalities, e.g. Marfan's (should correct values for body size and age), Ehlers–Danlos.
- First-degree relatives of people with myxomas (some rare familial forms associated with multiple freckles and HCM) or tuberous sclerosis.

2. Potential cardiac transplantation donors (on ITU) by TTE or TOE. The overall yield for conditions that eliminate the heart as a donor is approximately 1 in 4.
3. Baseline and follow-up re-evaluations of patients undergoing chemotherapy with cardiotoxic agents (e.g. doxorubicin, cumulative doses should be kept <450–500 mg/m^2).

Less clear-cut indications for screening echo

1. High risk of LV impairment
   - post-MI
   - alcohol excess
   - hypertension with LVH
   - LBBB in a young patient.
2. Systemic diseases that may affect the heart (see section 7.8).

'Follow-up' echo

This is performed in patients with some cardiac diseases at the intervals suggested below (more frequently if a clinical indication of deterioration such as development of new symptoms in previously controlled valve disease):

- Severe AS – 3–6 months
- Moderate AS – annual
- Moderate AR – 3–6 months
- HCM – annual
- Dilated aortic root – 6–12 months
- MV disease – annual
- Artificial biological valves – after 5 years then annual
- LV impairment – based on symptoms
- Following resection of cardiac tumour – annual for up to 5 years (recurrence rare).

7.7 ADVANCED AGE

There are predictable echo changes with advanced age:
- Progressive angulation between the descending aorta and the LVOT
- Localized proximal septal bulge resulting in a sigmoid shape to the proximal ventricular septum (upper septal bulge)
- Thickening of aortic wall
- Focal thickening of AV, MV and chordae
- MV annular calcification
- Increased myocardial stiffness causing diastolic function changes detected on pulsed wave Doppler as changes in the E to A ratio
- Mild LA dilatation
- A pattern mimicking HCM may develop, especially with hypertension that is poorly controlled.

7.8 ECHO ABNORMALITIES IN SOME SYSTEMIC DISEASES AND CONDITIONS

Some of these echo features may be present.

1. Infections

HIV infection and AIDS
- Dilated cardiomyopathy
- Myocarditis (e.g. due to opportunistic infections such as *Toxoplasma*, *Histoplasma*, cytomegalovirus)
- Pericardial effusion and tamponade
- Non-bacterial thrombotic endocarditis (marantic)
- Infective endocarditis (e.g. *Aspergillus*)
- Metastases from Kaposi's sarcoma
- PHT
- RV failure due to recurrent chest infections and PHT
- Effects of associated coronary disease.

Chagas' disease

This is caused by *Trypanosoma cruzi* and is endemic in Central and South America. It is one of the most common cause of heart failure worldwide with 20 million people affected.

- Myocarditis in acute stages
- Echo features similar to dilated cardiomyopathy
- Apical aneurysm common.

Lyme disease

This is caused by the tick-borne spirochaete *Borrelia burgdorferi.*
- Myocarditis, pericarditis
- LV dysfunction.

2. Inflammatory, rheumatic and connective tissue diseases

Marfan's syndrome (Fig. 7.2)

This is an autosomal dominant condition, so screen relatives (see section 7.6). Spontaneous mutation may occur in up to 30%.
- MV and TV prolapse
- Aortic root dilatation
- Aortic dissection
- Dilatation of sinus of Valsalva
- Endocarditis.

SLE

- Pericarditis and effusion
- Infective endocarditis
- Noninfective endocarditis (Libman–Sacks).

Rheumatoid arthritis

- Pericarditis and effusion, occasionally constriction
- Infiltration of rheumatoid nodules, valvular involvement causing regurgitation (aortic > mitral) (rare).

Ankylosing spondylitis

- Aortic root dilatation
- AV thickening
- AR
- Myocardial involvement.

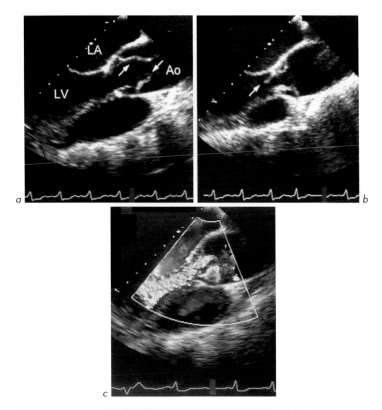

Fig. 7.2 *Marfan's syndrome. Dissecting aneurysm of ascending aorta. TOE study (aortic long-axis views).* **(a)** *The dissection flaps are seen (arrows).* **(b)** *There is prolapse of an aortic valve cusp (arrow).* **(c)** *Severe aortic regurgitation.*

Rheumatic heart disease

Acute rheumatic fever is very rare in Western countries but still common in developing countries.

- Myocarditis
- Endocarditis (valvulitis)
- Pericarditis
- Consequences – rheumatic valve disease years later.

3. Endocrine

Diabetes

- Effects of co-existent coronary disease or hypertension
- LV dysfunction – mild to severe, systolic (like dilated cardiomyopathy) or diastolic (of the 'restrictive type'), often in combination.

Acromegaly

- LVH, particularly of septum
- Dilated LV
- LV dysfunction
- Effects of co-existent coronary disease.

Hypothyroidism

- LVH
- LV or RV dilatation and systolic dysfunction, improve with treatment.

Hyperparathyroidism

- Valvular calcification related to hypercalcaemia – may lead rarely to stenosis or regurgitation.

4. Infiltrations

Amyloid

- LVH (concentric with a sparkling 'ground glass' appearance)
- Normal LV cavity until late in disease (when dilatation may occur)
- RV hypertrophy
- Hypertrophy of IAS
- Valvular thickening
- Dilated LA and RA
- LV diastolic dysfunction if advanced ('restrictive' mitral flow pattern with very high E-wave and a small A-wave)
- LV systolic dysfunction in advanced cases (poor prognosis)
- Pericardial effusion.

Sarcoid

- Bright IVS with normal or increased thickness and regions of thinning (scarring), especially at base of septum

- Involvement of papillary muscles
- Myocarditis
- Restrictive cardiomyopathy
- LV dilated with abnormal wall motion
- RV involvement
- LA dilatation
- MR and/or TR
- Diastolic or systolic impairment.

Haemochromatosis

In this condition, there is deposition of iron in many organs of the body. Idiopathic haemochromatosis is an autosomal recessive condition. The heart is involved in most advanced cases and the echo features are:

- Dilated cardiomyopathy pattern – dilated LV with reduced systolic function
- Infiltrative pattern (similar to amyloid) – LVH and abnormal myocardial texture.

5. Chronic anaemia (including haemoglobinopathies)

- LVH, usually eccentric
- LV dilatation
- LV diastolic dysfunction.

6. Hypertension

- LVH – may show regression on serial echo with treatment
- LV impairment
- Aortic dilatation
- Aortic dissection
- Effects of associated coronary artery disease.

7. Renal failure

- Pericardial effusion (uraemia)
- LV dysfunction (may improve with haemodialysis)
- Effects of co-existent coronary disease.

8. Malignancies

- Pericardial effusion
- Cardiac tumour due to direct invasion or metastasis
- Noninfective endocarditis (marantic).

9. Obesity

- This is associated with other cardiovascular risks and there may be echo features of hypertensive changes with LVH, changes related to coronary artery disease and diabetes mellitus.
- Morbid obesity – this is associated with a high output state and in extreme forms with congestive heart failure.
- Lesser degrees of obesity are associated with a slight increase in LV mass and internal dimensions and subtle systolic and diastolic dysfunction but usually there is a weak relationship when corrected for height and lean body mass.

10. Muscular dystrophies, dystrophia myotonica, Refsum's disease and Friedreich's ataxia

These genetic neuromuscular abnormalities can have cardiac effects. The echo features are of cardiomyopathies:

- Cardiac involvement typically mimics HCM or dilated cardiomyopathy.
- There may be regional variations in LV dysfunction.
- Duchenne muscular dystrophy and dystrophia myotonica – autosomal dominant conditions associated with cardiomyopathy.
- Refsum's disease (increased plasma phytanic acid due to defective lipid α-oxidase) is associated with a cardiomyopathy.
- Friedreich's ataxia (spinocerebellar degeneration, usually autosomal recessive) – the typical echo feature is a posterior LV wall motion abnormality.

11. Diet drug valvulopathies

Treatment with centrally-acting appetite suppressant (anorexic) drugs (especially a combination of fenfluramine and phentermine but also dexfenfluramine) has been associated with an unusual form of valve disease. This occurs in 3–15% of cases. The likelihood relates to the duration of treatment and is more likely to happen if the treatment is carried on for more than 6 months, although this is controversial. There are no universally agreed echo findings, and the changes may regress with time if treatment is discontinued. The echo features are:

- MV is most likely to be affected by a lesion. In advanced cases, the valve and chordae are encased in a matrix similar to that seen in carcinoid. This leads to MR. TV is spared.
- AR may occur but the echo appearances of the AV are normal.
- PHT may occur rarely.

Conclusions

- Many features of echo are explained by simple physiology.
- Echo can give important anatomical and functional information about the heart.
- Echo often influences the clinical management of a patient.
- Echo is a useful adjunct to the history and examination – *not* an alternative!

Further reading

ACC/AHA 1997 ACC/AHA guidelines for the clinical application of echocardiography. Circulation 95:1686–1744

Asmi M H, Walsh M J 1998 A practical guide to echocardiography. Hodder Arnold, London

Bax J J, Abraham S, Barold O, et al 2005 Cardiac resynchronization therapy: Part 1 – issues before device implantation. Journal of the American College of Cardiology 46:2153–2167

Bax J J, Abraham S, Barold O, et al 2005 Cardiac resynchronization therapy: Part 2 – issues during and after device implantation and unresolved questions. Journal of the American College of Cardiology 46:2168–2182

Chambers J B 1995 Clinical echocardiography. BMJ Publications, London

Chambers J B 1996 Echocardiography in primary care. Parthenon, London

Cheitlin M D, Armstrong W F, Aurigemma G P et al; ACC/AHA/ASE 2003 Guideline update for the clinical application of echocardiography: summary article: a report of the American College of Cardiology/American Heart Association Task Force on Practice Guidelines (ACC/AHA/ASE Committee to Update the 1997 Guidelines for the Clinical Application of Echocardiography). Circulation 108:1146–1162

Dobb G J 2003 Cardiogenic shock. In: Bersten A, Soni N, Oh T E (eds) Oh's intensive care manual, 5th edn. Butterworth-Heinemann, Oxford

Eagle K A, Berger P B, Calkins H, et al; American College of Cardiology/American Heart Association Task Force on Practice Guidelines (Committee to Update the 1996 Guidelines on Perioperative Cardiovascular Evaluation for Noncardiac Surgery) 2002 ACC/AHA guideline update for perioperative cardiovascular evaluation for noncardiac surgery – executive summary of a report of the American College of Cardiology/American Heart Association Task Force on Practice Guidelines (Committee to Update the 1996 Guidelines on Perioperative Cardiovascular Evaluation for Noncardiac Surgery). Circulation 105(10):1257–1267

European Society of Cardiology 2007 Guidelines for cardiac pacing and cardiac resynchronization therapy: the task force for cardiac resynchronization therapy of the European Society of Cardiology. European Heart Journal 28:2256–2295

Everbach E C 2007 Medical diagnostic ultrasound. Physics Today March: 44–48

Feigenbaum H 2005 Echocardiography, 6th edn. Lea & Febiger, Philadelphia

Focus issue 2005 Cardiac resynchronization therapy. Journal of the American College of Cardiology 46:2153–2367

Holmberg S 1996 Acute heart failure. In: Julian D G, Camm A J, Fox K M, Hall R J C, et al (eds) Diseases of the heart, 2nd edn. W B Saunders, London, p 456–466

Hung J, Lang R, Flachskampf F, et al 2007 3D echocardiography: a review of the current status and future directions. Journal of the American Society of Echocardiography 20:213–233

Kaddoura S, Oldershaw P J 1994 Pulmonary vascular disease and management of the Eisenmenger reaction. In: Redington A, Shore D, Oldershaw P J (eds) A practical guide to congenital heart disease in adults. W B Saunders, London, p 213–228

Kaddoura S, Poole-Wilson P A 1999 Acute heart failure. In: Dalla Volta S, de Bayes Luna A, Brochier M, et al (eds) Cardiology. McGraw-Hill, Milan, p 517–521

Kaddoura S, Poole-Wilson P A 1999 Cardiogenic shock. In: Dalla Volta S, de Bayes Luna A, Brochier M, et al (eds) Cardiology. McGraw-Hill, Milan, p 535–541

Kaddoura S, Poole-Wilson P A 1999 Chronic heart failure. In: Dalla Volta S, de Bayes Luna A, Brochier M, et al (eds) Cardiology. McGraw-Hill, Milan, p 523–533

Kremkau F W 2007 Seeing is believing? Sonographic artefacts. Physics Today March: 84–85

Monaghan M J 1990 Practical echocardiography and Doppler. John Wiley, Chichester

NICE 2007 Technology appraisal guidance 120. Cardiac resynchronization therapy for the treatment of heart failure. Online. Available: www.nice.org.uk/TA120

Otto C M 2004 Textbook of clinical echocardiography, 3rd edn. Elsevier Science, Philadelphia

Otto C M 2007 The practice of clinical echocardiography, 3rd edn. Saunders, London

Physics Today 2007 Focus on ultrasound. March 2007. American Institute of Physics

St John Sutton M G, Oldershaw P J, Kotler M N (eds) 1996 Textbook of echocardiography and Doppler in adults and children, 2nd edn. Blackwell Science, Cambridge, MA

Sutherland G R, Roelandt J R T C, Fraser A G, Anderson R H 1991 Transoesophageal echocardiography in clinical practice. Gower Medical, London

Swanton R H 2003 Cardiology, 5th edn. Blackwell Science, Oxford

Winter S, Nesser H J 2007 Echocardiography for cardiac resynchronization. The next step. Medtronic, Vienna

Zipes D P, Libby P, Bonow R O, Braunwald E 2004 Braunwald's heart disease. A textbook of cardiovascular medicine, 7th edn. W B Saunders, Philadelphia

Websites providing useful guidelines

www.acc.org/qualityandscience/clinical/statements.htm
www.americanheart.org/presenter.jhtml?identifier=3004612
www.asecho.org/Guidelines.php
www.escardio.org/knowledge/guidelines
www.nice.org.uk

Index

W